P9-DCR-431

What women have to say after trying the LEVITY program:

"I lost 5 pounds, and I wasn't really on a diet!"

"I have a lot more energy."

"I no longer feel like I'm on the edge of 'losing it.'"

"I wake up refreshed, not worried."

"My husband says I look much healthier."

"Sex is more enjoyable now."

When Your Body Gets The Blues

The Clinically Proven Program for Women Who Feel Tired and Stressed and Eat Too Much

Marie-Annette Brown, Ph.D., R.N., and Jo Robinson

RODALE

Notice

This book is intended as a reference volume only, not as a medical manual. The information given here is designed to help you make informed decisions about your health. It is not intended as a substitute for any treatment that may have been prescribed by your doctor. If you suspect that you have a medical problem, we urge you to seek competent medical help.

Mention of specific companies, organizations, or authorities in this book does not imply endorsement by the publisher, nor does mention of specific companies, organizations, or authorities in the book imply that they endorse the book.

Internet addresses and telephone numbers given in this book were accurate at the time it went to press.

© 2002 by Marie-Annette Brown, Ph.D., and Jo Robinson
Cover photograph © Derek P. Redfearn/The Image Bank

All rights reserved. No part of this publication may be reproduced or transmitted in any form or by any means, electronic or mechanical, including photocopying, recording, or any other information storage and retrieval system, without the written permission of the publisher.

Printed in the United States of America
Rodale Inc. makes every effort to use acid-free ∞, recycled paper ♻.

"The Effects of a Multi-Modal Intervention Trial of Light, Exercise, and Vitamins on Women's Mood" on page 172 is reprinted with permission from *Women and Health*, vol. 34, no. 3. © 2001 The Haworth Press, Binghamton, New York.

Interior design by Darlene Schneck
Cover design by Carol Angstadt
Graph and chart design by Christina Gaugler

Library of Congress Cataloging-in-Publication Data

Brown, Marie-Annette.
When your body gets the blues : the clinically proven program for women who feel tired and stressed and eat too much / Marie-Annette Brown and Jo Robinson.
        p.   cm.
Includes bibliographical references and index.
ISBN 1–57954–486–X   hardcover
1. Depression in women—Popular works.   2. Women—Health and hygiene.   3. Stress management for women.   I. Robinson, Jo, date.   II. Title.
RC537 .B763   2002
616.85'27'0082—dc21   2001006285

Distributed to the book trade by St. Martin's Press

2   4   6   8   10   9   7   5   3   1   hardcover

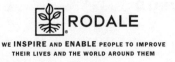

RODALE
WE **INSPIRE** AND **ENABLE** PEOPLE TO IMPROVE
THEIR LIVES AND THE WORLD AROUND THEM

FOR MORE OF OUR PRODUCTS
WWW.RODALESTORE.COM
(800) 848-4735

Contents

PART 3: How to Follow the LEVITY Program

PART 4: Resources and References

Acknowledgments

Successful research requires dedication and teamwork. Jo Robinson and I are deeply grateful to the 112 women who invested their precious time to conscientiously participate in all the activities required to test the LEVITY program. Equally essential was the hard work and commitment of the University of Washington School of Nursing LEVITY research team—Susan M. Casey, Ph.C., M.S., R.N.; Ann Frolich, M.N., F.N.P.; Jamie Goldstein-Shirley, Ph.C., M.S.N., R.N.; Crista Langstrom, M.N., F.N.P.; Kathy Pearce, M.N., F.N.P.; and Vernetta Stewart, M.N., P.S.N.P. Their enthusiasm, creativity, and collaborative spirit helped us conduct a successful study despite our limited funding. We are particularly grateful for the leadership and organizational and analytic skills of Jamie Goldstein-Shirley, doctoral candidate in nursing, who tirelessly served as project manager and creatively enhanced our design and analysis as a co-investigator and creator of this intervention trial.

We are also deeply grateful for the encouragement and assistance of my University of Washington colleagues as we carried out this challenging and all-consuming research project that included months of analysis and writing. My special thanks to my department chairs, Marcia Killien, Ph.D., R.N., F.A.A.N., and Kristen Swanson, Ph.D., R.N., F.A.A.N. I also want to acknowledge the help and support of the administrators and staff at the Women's Center, especially Emily Wong, M.D., and Grace Parker, M.N., R.N. Our special thanks to Frances Robinson, our "pre-editor," who enabled us to present a manuscript to our editors at Rodale that required little additional work.

We are indebted to our agent, Richard Pine, for his expertise in conceiving and marketing health books. Richard helped shape *When Your Body Gets the Blues* from its inception and found it a happy home at Rodale.

At Rodale, we want to give special thanks to Tammerly Booth, editor-in-chief; Sharon Faelten, our patient and insightful senior editor; Karen Neely, our enthusiastic line editor; and Cindy Ratzlaff, executive director of publicity. We enjoyed very much working with these particular women and also with a publishing company that places a high premium on healthy people and a healthy planet.

We want to acknowledge the Center for Women's Health Research at the University of Washington and the Psi Chapter of Sigma Theta Tau, the nursing honorary society, for providing key financial support for the LEVITY study.

Finally, we wish to acknowledge our beloved family members and friends for their unflagging support and encouragement.

—Marie-Annette Brown, Ph.D., R.N., and Jo Robinson

PART 1

The Problem

Chapter 1

The Body Blues
Women's Number One Mood Problem

At any given time, tens of millions of women are troubled by a syndrome for which they have no name. One of the most common complaints is feeling tired and sluggish much of the time. To their dismay, the women don't have enough energy to be the patient moms, supportive partners, or fun-loving friends they would like to be. Although they know that exercise would help revive them, they rarely have both the time and the motivation.

Many women with this syndrome have sleep difficulties as well. They have trouble falling asleep or staying asleep—or they sleep too much. The common denominator is that they feel drowsy during the day, whether due to a lack of sleep or general drowsiness. Those times when they feel alert and energetic all day long are a welcome relief.

Difficulty concentrating is another telltale sign of this disorder, especially in women 35 and older. The women have trouble focusing on tasks, absorbing complex information, or finding just the right words to say when they talk. Verbal slips and difficulty remembering names—even the names of people they know really well—can be a source of embarrassment. Curiously, these mental lapses can come and go. For days at a time, they feel mentally sharp. Then, for some unknown reason, their thinking becomes fuzzy or scattered. It's as though their IQs had dropped 10 points overnight. Middle-aged women can be especially troubled by these mental symptoms because they fear they might have the early signs of Alzheimer's disease.

Many of the women also feel stressed and irritable. They can be annoyed by simple things such as the sound of construction from a neighbor's house, a partner's eating habits, or being put on hold on the phone. Even when the pressure is off, some women find it hard to relax. A drink or two is a fast way to unwind, but relying on alcohol to relax can lead to alcohol dependency. A more common way to relieve stress is to watch TV or read a book. These two remedies work reasonably well, but they take away from the little time women have to be creative or take on ambitious projects.

But the most common and vexing symptoms of this syndrome are overeating and weight gain. In the morning, most of the women have little trouble controlling their appetite. But sometime in the afternoon, they begin to snack. They also feel an urge to eat whenever they are feeling anxious, tired, or stressed. Women say that certain foods are more soothing than others, especially pasta, pizza, sweets, bread, and chocolate. In fact, a craving for sweets and starches is one of the defining characteristics of this syndrome.

The logical result of feeling too tired to exercise and eating too much is being overweight. Some women manage to keep the pounds off through rigorous dieting, but most plateau at a high weight or continue to gain weight year after year. One reason being overweight is so troubling to them is that they can't cover it up. If need be, they can disguise the fact that they're sleeping poorly, forgetting names, or feeling irritable. But they can't deny that they're overweight. It's the one visible sign of their distress.

There's another symptom that one might expect to find on this list—a depressed mood. But women who have this syndrome do not have serious mood problems. Unlike women with clinical depression, they do not feel sad or tearful all the time. They don't feel hopeless or think that the world would be a better place without them. When something good happens to them, they feel genuinely happy. Most of them perform well at work, even those with high-level, demanding jobs. Nonetheless, they can be very distressed by their fatigue, eating problems, irritability, confused thinking, or sleep difficulties. These symptoms interfere with their relationships, frustrate their ambitions, and rob them of the full enjoyment of life. It's as though their *bodies* were depressed, but not their minds. They have what I call the "Body Blues."

What Is the Body Blues?

The textbook term for the Body Blues is *vegetative depressive symptoms*.[1] A woman with this condition has three or more of the symptoms listed below to such a degree that they diminish her enjoyment in life and sense of well-being.

- Eating too much and gaining weight
- Low energy

- Difficulty concentrating
- Sleep difficulties
- Irritability or tension
- Daytime drowsiness
- Decreased interest in sex
- Mild anxiety
- Mild depression
- Heightened sensitivity to rejection or criticism

A woman can have the Body Blues all by itself, or it can be a part of other disorders. For example, PMS could be viewed as the Body Blues plus bloating, cramps, or breast tenderness. Postpartum depression, or the "baby blues," could be seen as the Body Blues but with more severe mood problems. Menopausal symptoms could be characterized as the Body Blues plus hot flashes and physical signs of aging. Seasonal affective disorder (SAD), also known as winter depression, could be regarded as a seasonal siege of the Body Blues. Embedded in all these disorders is the same core group of symptoms listed above.

Men can have symptoms of the Body Blues as well, especially those 40 or older. But the syndrome is far more common in women. First of all, most of the disorders that include symptoms of the Body Blues, such as PMS and the baby blues, are exclusive to women. But even the unisex disorders, such as SAD, are three or more times as common in women as men. For reasons I will explore in more depth in chapter 2, the Body Blues seems to go hand in hand with being female.

Joanne: A Portrait of the Body Blues

In addition to being a professor and researcher at the University of Washington School of Nursing, I am a primary care provider for female patients at the university's Women's Health Care Clinic. Like most practitioners, I see a steady stream of women with the Body Blues. One of my patients (I'll call her "Joanne") has four of the most common symptoms—fatigue, irritability, low sexual desire, and weight gain. Although these problems bother her a great deal, few people would sense that anything is wrong with her. To the casual observer, she appears to be a competent, confident woman who happens to be slightly overweight.

The primary reason that Joanne made the initial appointment is that she feels tired much of the time. On most nights, she gets 7 to 8 hours of sleep, but when she wakes up in the morning, she still does not feel refreshed. By early afternoon, she is overwhelmed by the need to take a nap. Because her office is in her home, she can lie down whenever she needs to, but she resents taking the time. Napping also makes her feel lazy. "I'm only 39," she told me, "I shouldn't have to take a nap! I feel like my grandmother! Before I had employees, I could nap and not feel guilty. Now I have to sneak around to get the rest that I need."

Joanne also feels stressed and irritable much of the time. "My family bears the brunt of it," she told me. "My employees and clients soak up most of my patience during the day. My son gets what's left. My husband—I'm much more critical of him than I want to be. And for about 5 years, I've had much less interest in sex. Once I get aroused, I enjoy sex. I say, 'Hey, Jim! That felt really good! Why don't we do this more often?' But when I'm not making love, I have little interest in sex at all. Most nights, I'd rather read a book."

Even though Joanne listed fatigue as her reason for making the appointment, I could see that she was even more concerned about her weight. At 5 feet 6 and 172 pounds, she is about 30 pounds overweight. "I have no problem controlling what I eat for breakfast and lunch," she told me during that first appointment, "but everything falls apart in the late afternoon. I eat before dinner, during dinner, and after dinner. It's like I'm on a diet for the first half of the day, then I blow it the second half. I do this day after day." The net result of her frequent snacking and low energy is that she has been gaining about a pound or two every month. Even though she is not obese, her weight troubles her a great deal. She is unhappy about how she looks and feels ashamed that she can't tame her appetite. "I know everything there is to know about losing weight," she said. "I've done it dozens of times. But I can't keep it off. When I've dieted myself out of my size 16 clothes, I've learned not to throw them away because I know I'll be needing them again in a few months. Right now, I'm back in my fat clothes."

Although Joanne did not seem to be seriously depressed, I asked her some general questions about her mood just to make sure. She said her mood wasn't great, but she didn't think she was depressed. "I have my ups and downs," she said. "But most of the time, I feel okay."

"How do you feel about yourself?" I continued. "Do you often feel worthless or inadequate?" Many women have low self-esteem, but it is very common in women with serious mood disorders. Joanne laughed. "My husband would say I have the opposite problem—grandiosity. Most of the time, I'm pretty high on myself." Then she paused. "Except for being so tired. And my weight.

I can't seem to do anything about that. And the fact that I'm such a slob. My house is a mess. So is the car. I can haul four sacks of groceries into the house, but I don't go back that one last time to clean out the car. That bugs Jim to no end. When I drive his car, I clean it up. But I leave mine a mess."

As I listened to Joanne, it seemed that she had high self-esteem except when it came to the symptoms of the Body Blues. She thought she was overweight because she lacked willpower. She had a messy house because she was a "slob." I find some measure of self-blame in virtually all women with this syndrome. "Why can't I stick to a diet?" "I know I should exercise. Why don't I do it?" "Why can other women keep the weight off?" "My husband eats everything in the house, and he's not overweight." "Why am I so tired all the time?" "Why do I have so little interest in sex?" "Why can't I remember the names of my best friend's children?" In addition to being troubled by their vegetative symptoms, these women are weighed down by feelings of shame and blame. In some of my patients, the self-criticism seems just as burdensome as the symptoms themselves. Very few women realize that their eating problems and feelings of fatigue, stress, and irritability are due, in part, to their biology.

I asked Joanne if her symptoms got worse just before menstruation, and she said that they did. "But I don't feel great the rest of the month," she said. "It's just that I eat more and feel more tired and irritable just before my period." Normally, I would have asked if her symptoms were confined to the winter, indicating that she might have SAD. But this was the end of June, and she was still feeling sluggish and eating too much. People with SAD feel much better in the summer.

Finally, I asked her some questions about her diet, exercise habits, family relationships, and social support system. As a nurse practitioner, I've been trained to look at the whole person, not just her symptoms. I noted nothing in Joanne's responses that suggested she was in need of personal, marital, or family therapy. At the end of the appointment, I ordered some blood tests to make sure that she did not have any of the physical problems linked with fatigue such as an underactive thyroid, diabetes, mononucleosis, hepatitis, or anemia. A few days later, when all her tests came back negative, I was not surprised. As I had begun to suspect during her first appointment, Joanne is one of the millions of women with the Body Blues.

Why Is This Syndrome News?

The fact that women are prone to having this particular cluster of symptoms has been known for a long time. For example, in the 19th century, the

Body Blues was called "neurotic" or "nervous" depression and was considered a "female problem." The Victorians blamed this disorder on a woman's fragile constitution, her childlike nature, or her willful deviation from traditional femininity. Women at highest risk were thought to be those who were too involved in intellectual matters.

The 19th-century cures for the Body Blues seem just as foreign from our modern point of view. When a woman had problems with fatigue, for example, she was said to be "off her feet" and could be sent to bed for weeks on end. While sequestered in her dark room, she was to avoid having company or stimulating her mind—a cure that was in reality a recipe for depression! If a woman ate too much, she was said to be "eating like a ploughman." To tame her appetite, she might be subjected to bloodletting or leeches. If that didn't work, then her ovaries might be removed. Women who felt irritable or displayed "cussedness" were treated with laudanum—an addictive elixir of opium, sherry wine, and herbs guaranteed to cure anyone's ills.

Today, the Victorian remedies for the Body Blues and the 19th-century terms for the disorder are safely tucked away in the history books. The psychiatric community has chosen the label *vegetative depressive symptoms* because people who have this disorder tend to feel slowed down, weighed down, and sleepy, and they eat too much. In other words, they seem to "vegetate." The modern slang term "to veg out" has many of these same connotations. By contrast, people with more "typical" symptoms of depression have little appetite and tend to *lose* weight—the opposite of the Body Blues.

Until the 1990s, however, vegetative symptoms of depression were given scant attention. They were regarded as just another variety of depression that happened to be more common in women than men. Few people were aware that these symptoms could plague women throughout their reproductive years—first manifesting themselves as PMS, then as winter depression, followed by the baby blues, and then perimenopausal and menopausal symptoms. People were too busy focusing on each of these disorders as a separate entity to see what they all had in common.

The Prozac Phenomenon

One phenomenon in particular highlighted the similarities between these conditions—the widespread use of Prozac, the popular antidepressant medication introduced in 1988. Prozac was the first in a family of antidepressant drugs designed to boost the activity of serotonin, the brain's primary feel-good chemical. This family of drugs is referred to as selective serotonin re-uptake inhibitors, or SSRIs. Prozac proved to be just as good at treating depression as earlier medications, but with fewer side effects. Because the drug was so well-tolerated, researchers began to see whether it could treat other disorders as well.

Starting in the mid-1990s, Prozac and other SSRIs were given to people with a wide variety of conditions—including sleep problems, anxiety, obesity, bulimia, fatigue, chronic pain syndrome, fibromyalgia, SAD, and PMS—as well as to women going through perimenopause or menopause.[2] Surprisingly, the SSRIs helped relieve all of these seemingly unrelated problems. To the researchers, this suggested that a deficiency of serotonin must be one of their hidden causes. There was another factor that united all of these conditions—they were either exclusive to women or far more common in women than men. Did this mean that women are more likely than men to be deficient in serotonin?

The Estrogen-Serotonin Connection

It now appears that the answer is yes. Before the 1990s, researchers found little difference in the amount of serotonin in the bloodstream of men and women. But as scientists learned more about brain chemicals in general and serotonin in particular, they began to discover some very important differences between the sexes. For example, men and women differ in the number and effectiveness of the receptors that grab on to serotonin and make it available to the brain cells.[3] This means that a man and woman could have the same amount of serotonin in their brains, but men would make better use of the mood-elevating chemical.

An even more important discovery, however, is that the serotonin activity in a woman's brain ebbs and flows with her production of estrogen.[4] When women have high estrogen levels, they have more serotonin activity in their brains. When they have low or falling estrogen levels, they have less serotonin activity.

When do women have low or falling levels of estrogen? They are most likely to have low or declining estrogen production (1) in the days before menstruation, (2) after giving birth, (3) while breastfeeding, (4) during perimenopause, and (5) during all the decades following menopause. These happen to be the very times when women are most likely to have vegetative symptoms of depression. One could almost say that low estrogen equals low serotonin equals the Body Blues.

Women, Stress, and Serotonin

There's one more occasion when women are more likely to be deficient in serotonin than men—during periods of prolonged stress. It's been known for a number of years that when people are under stress, they go through their store of serotonin at a faster pace, requiring their brain cells to speed up production. But a startling new finding is that women may replenish their supply of this feel-good chemical more slowly than men.

In a 1997 study, investigators used a sophisticated imaging technique called positron emission tomography, or PET, to peer inside the brains of male and female volunteers. The PET scans showed that the men were producing serotonin 50 percent faster than the women.[5] Years ago, the fact that women might have a larger corpus callosum—the bridge between the right and left hemispheres of their brains—was the topic of much discussion. The new finding that men produce nature's antidepressant more rapidly than women could prove to be a much more significant discovery.

Hampered with a slower production of serotonin, a woman becomes vulnerable to the Body Blues when she is under prolonged stress. Imagine, for a moment, a situation in which a woman and her husband are subjected to the very same stressful situation. Let's suppose that they receive a registered letter from the IRS saying that they have underpaid their taxes for 5 years and may be facing penalties and criminal charges. Once the initial panic subsides, the couple endures weeks of anxiety and pressure as they spend long hours with their tax lawyer, stay up late going through their financial records, and worry about the possible criminal charges. The constant stress uses up their serotonin at a faster-than-normal pace. But the woman makes up for the deficiency more slowly than her husband, making her deficient in serotonin for more of the time. When the matter with the IRS is finally resolved, it's not surprising that she has gained a considerable amount of weight and feels more stressed and depressed than her husband: She has been handicapped by a slower production of serotonin.

A Syndrome in Search of a Cure

If one of the underlying causes of the Body Blues is low serotonin activity, then the obvious solution is for women to take drugs that boost this essential brain chemical. Hundreds of thousands of women are now following this course of action. But none of the medications now on the market is a comprehensive solution for the Body Blues. Typically, the drugs help with some symptoms but make others worse. For example, a drug that makes a woman feel happier and more energetic can interfere with her ability to have orgasms. Or a medication that tames a woman's appetite can make her feel jittery and disrupt her sleep. Or a drug that helps calm a woman's anxiety can cause her to gain weight—a side effect few women will tolerate.

When one of my patients is seriously depressed or her symptoms are interfering with her ability to function, I recommend the use of appropriate medications. For some of my patients, antidepressants have proven to be life-saving. But the Body Blues is not a life-threatening mood disorder. The syndrome is burdensome and annoying and erodes a woman's sense of well-being, but it is not a severe condition. Many of my patients with this syndrome have come to the same understanding. When I discuss various treatment options with them, including SSRIs, one of the most common refrains is "I'm not all that depressed." Other women have a strong preference for relieving their symptoms in a more natural way. They say to me, "I don't want to solve my problems with a prescription drug."

In search of a more natural solution, many women turn to alternative remedies for relief. There are now hundreds of products on the market that promise to cure some aspect of the Body Blues. There are teas, tinctures, and supplements that promise to enhance your mood, help you lose weight, improve your memory, calm your anxiety, spark your sexual desire, or help you sleep like a baby. Because women with the Body Blues tend to have a number of these symptoms, some take a handful of supplements each day.

I am open to the use of herbal treatments or dietary supplements in general. Some show signs of living up to their claims and have fewer side effects than prescription drugs. But many of the products now on the market have not been adequately tested for their effectiveness, quality, or safety. And there is some concern as to whether they even contain the amount of active ingredients specified on their labels. Even when the products contain the right ingredients in the advertised amounts, many women don't get the relief they are seeking. They try one remedy for a few weeks and then discard it for the newest and latest herbal cure. Or they keep taking the old products and add a new one on top of them. As one of my patients confided, "I don't know if any of them is working, so I take them all."

As a rough estimate, I would guess that about one quarter of the millions of women with the Body Blues seek relief from antidepressants and another

Herbal Roulette

"EACH DAY, I TAKE five or six different pills. I take ginseng for fatigue, ginkgo biloba for my memory, L-arginine for my sex drive, kava kava for anxiety, and valerian to help me sleep. I don't like taking so many pills, but at least they're not antidepressants or heart medications. They're all natural."

LEVITY volunteer, 48

quarter turn to alternative remedies. But, sadly, the rest of the women do nothing at all for their vegetative symptoms. Many do not know that they have a treatable disorder, so they simply do their best to cope. Some are ashamed of their symptoms, so they don't make an appointment to discuss them with their health care practitioners. Typically, I first learn that one of my patients has vegetative symptoms when I ask general health questions during her annual cervical and breast exam. If I didn't know what to look for and which questions to ask, I would never know she is troubled by the Body Blues.

But even when women go to their health care practitioners specifically to talk about their vegetative symptoms, many do not get the help they deserve. One problem is that many health professionals focus only on the physical causes of a woman's mood symptoms. When the lab tests come back negative, they give her a clean bill of health. Other practitioners do not view mild depression as a significant problem. They've been trained to focus on symptoms of major depression, such as a loss of pleasure in most activities, thoughts of death, feelings of worthlessness, reduced interest in food, and unexplained weight loss. Milder vegetative symptoms such as fatigue, overeating, and weight gain fail to register on their radar screens.

A separate issue is that few of the tests that doctors use to screen their patients for depression are designed to detect the common symptoms of the Body Blues. For example, one of the most frequently used tests in general practice is called the Beck Depression Inventory, or BDI. The BDI asks you if you have noticed a decrease in appetite and recent weight loss—but not if you've been eating more and putting on weight. If the BDI included these two vegetative symptoms, most women would score higher, sending a clear signal that they warrant some form of treatment.

For all of these reasons—(1) the lack of a comprehensive, effective therapy; (2) women's hesitancy to talk about their mood problems; (3) the failure of health professionals to look for vegetative depressive symptoms; and (4) the lack of appropriate diagnostic tools—*the Body Blues is women's most misdiagnosed, undertreated, and mistreated mood problem.*

The LEVITY Program: The Clinically Proven Solution to the Body Blues

My colleagues and I at the University of Washington spent several years tackling the first of these problems—the lack of an effective, appropriate therapy for the Body Blues. Our goal was to develop a therapy that is drug-free and inexpensive and that removes the underlying causes of the syndrome rather than simply treating the symptoms. We also wanted the program to be genuinely helpful to women of all ages, employment statuses, and walks of life. This meant that it would have to require very little time, be inherently enjoyable, and be suitable for women of all levels of physical fitness. As women and nurse practitioners, we were acutely aware of the realities of women's lives. Finally, because we also wanted the program to be prescribed by a multitude of busy health professionals, we knew that it would also have to be rigorously tested and easy to administer.

As you will learn in more detail later on, the therapy we developed and tested is based on three commonsense activities.

- Creating a more natural lighting environment
- Going for a 20-minute, brisk outdoor walk, five or more times a week
- Taking six common and inexpensive vitamins and minerals

In a light-hearted moment, my colleagues and I dubbed this therapy "the LEVITY program," with LEVITY being a tortured acronym for **L**ight, **E**xercise, and **V**itamin **I**ntervention Therap**Y**. We tested the program on 112 mildly depressed women spanning the ages of 19 to 78. All of them had vegetative symptoms of depression. We randomly assigned the women to one of two groups. One group was given placebo vitamins with no other form of treatment and served as the "control" group. The other group took part in all three activities of the LEVITY program.

Before and after the 8-week study, we gave the women five standardized tests to see if the program had relieved their symptoms. In a consistency rarely seen in studies of this nature, the women who took part in the program improved significantly more than the women who took placebo pills on every one of the tests. In particular, they had:

✓ Fewer eating and weight problems
✓ More vitality
✓ Less anxiety

✓ Less anger
✓ Better self-esteem
✓ More self-control
✓ Less irritability
✓ Less tension

The program had reduced virtually all the symptoms of the Body Blues! Just as important, it had greatly enhanced the women's moods. On one of the standardized tests, the women's average depression score was cut in half.[6] This is comparable to the effects of some well-known antidepressants. Yet the program was free of negative side effects and cost just pennies a day.

When we completed our analysis of the data, we submitted our findings to the journal *Women and Health*.[7] After careful peer review, the paper was accepted for publication in 2001. You will find a reprint of the article on page 172 of this book.

Do You Have the Body Blues?

Although the Body Blues is very common among women, not every woman has it. My best guess is that one out of every four women has the syndrome at any given time.[8] To see whether or not you have this disorder, I invite you to take the comprehensive quiz that follows.

If your scores show that you do have the Body Blues, you will be pleased to know that this book contains all the instructions and support you need to enjoy the clinically proven benefits of the LEVITY program. The vitamins and minerals are inexpensive and available at most supermarkets. (If you wish, you can also purchase the same tablets we used in our study. See page 160 for ordering information.) The only equipment you'll need is a comfortable pair of walking shoes. In a few weeks, you will be enjoying the same results as the women in our study. You will be eating less, feeling more energetic, coping better with stress, feeling more upbeat, and finding more enjoyment in your everyday life. Best of all, you will have achieved these results through your own efforts.

The Body Blues Quiz

This quiz has three sections. Answer the questions in each section in terms of how you've been feeling during the *past few weeks*. Write down the number of points associated with each answer in the space provided.

Section A

In the past few weeks . . .

1. I've been feeling tired or sluggish.
   ❒ Not at all (0) ❒ Occasionally (1) ❒ Often (2) ❒ Most of the time (3)
   _____Points

2. I've been having difficulty falling asleep or staying asleep.
   ❒ Not at all (0) ❒ Occasionally (1) ❒ Often (2) ❒ Most of the time (3)
   _____Points

3. I've been eating more than I would like, especially in the second half of the day.
   ❒ Not at all (0) ❒ Occasionally (1) ❒ Often (2) ❒ Most of the time (3)
   _____Points

4. My thinking has seemed fuzzy or unfocused.
   ❒ Not at all (0) ❒ Occasionally (1) ❒ Often (2) ❒ Most of the time (3)
   _____Points

5. I've had little interest in sex.
   ❒ Not at all (0) ❒ Occasionally (1) ❒ Often (2) ❒ Most of the time (3)
   _____Points

6. I've been feeling tense or anxious.
   ❒ Not at all (0) ❒ Occasionally (1) ❒ Often (2) ❒ Most of the time (3)
   _____Points

7. I've had difficulty coping with stress.
   ❒ Not at all (0) ❒ Occasionally (1) ❒ Often (2) ❒ Most of the time (3)
   _____Points

8. I've been feeling drowsy or sleepy in the afternoons.
   ❒ Not at all (0) ❒ Occasionally (1) ❒ Often (2) ❒ Most of the time (3)
   _____Points

9. I've been craving sweets, chocolate, or carbohydrates.
   ❒ Not at all (0) ❒ Occasionally (1) ❒ Often (2) ❒ Most of the time (3)
   _____Points

10. I've been thinking about death in general, my own mortality, or losing others.
    ❒ Not at all (0) ❒ Occasionally (1) ❒ Often (2) ❒ Most of the time (3)
    _____Points

11. I've been eating when I feel tired, irritable, anxious, or sad.
    ❐ Not at all (0)   ❐ Occasionally (1)   ❐ Often (2)   ❐ Most of the time (3)
    _____Points

12. I've been feeling the urge to buy things to boost my mood.
    ❐ Not at all (0)   ❐ Occasionally (1)   ❐ Often (2)   ❐ Most of the time (3)
    _____Points

13. I've been feeling irritable or angry.
    ❐ Not at all (0)   ❐ Occasionally (1)   ❐ Often (2)   ❐ Most of the time (3)
    _____Points

14. I've been making "verbal slips" or having difficulty recalling names or choosing just the right word.
    ❐ Not at all (0)   ❐ Occasionally (1)   ❐ Often (2)   ❐ Most of the time (3)
    _____Points

15. I've been having problems making decisions.
    ❐ Not at all (0)   ❐ Occasionally (1)   ❐ Often (2)   ❐ Most of the time (3)
    _____Points

16. I've been snacking after dinner.
    ❐ Not at all (0)   ❐ Occasionally (1)   ❐ Often (2)   ❐ Most of the time (3)
    _____Points

Add up all your points in section A and write the number here:_____

Section B

In the past few weeks . . .

1. I've had a greatly diminished interest or pleasure in all, or almost all, activities.
   ❐ Not at all (0)   ❐ Occasionally (1)   ❐ Often (2)   ❐ Most of the time (3)
   _____Points

2. I've been very depressed, sad, tearful, or feeling flat.
   ❐ Not at all (0)   ❐ Occasionally (1)   ❐ Often (2)   ❐ Most of the time (3)
   _____Points

3. I've been feeling so low or depressed that I've had a very hard time functioning.
   ❐ Not at all (0)   ❐ Occasionally (1)   ❐ Often (2)   ❐ Most of the time (3)
   _____Points

Total points in section B:_____

Section C

In the past few weeks . . .

1. I have been wishing I were dead or thinking about ways I might take my own life.
   ❐ Yes
   ❐ No

STOP HERE. If you responded yes to this final statement, I strongly urge you to seek help, either from your primary care provider or a mental health professional. Make sure that you give a full and accurate reporting of your symptoms. Many depressed people hesitate to reveal how bad they feel. With the proper care, you are likely to feel better in a matter of weeks. Then you can add the LEVITY program to more conventional treatments.

If you answered no to this question, proceed to the flow chart on the next page.

Questions and Answers about the Quiz

Q. I scored very high in section A—39 points out of 48 possible points. I'm wondering if the LEVITY program will help me enough.

A. Interestingly, the women in our study who were the most depressed and anxious improved significantly more than those who had milder mood problems. If you do not feel noticeably better in 2 to 3 weeks, however, I recommend that you make an appointment with your health care provider.

Q. I scored 5 points in section B, indicating that I might have serious depression. Should I try the program first before I seek help?

A. We did not test our program on women with major depression, so we don't know if the program meets the needs of people with more serious mood disorders. You can try the program for a few weeks to see if it makes a noticeable difference. If you have been thinking about your own death, however, or cannot carry out your normal activities or are experiencing a great deal of anguish, I urge that you see a health care professional now. You can always add the LEVITY program to more conventional forms of treatment.

Q. My scores were low (7 points in section A and 0 points in B), but I would like to try the program anyway. Will I see any change?

A. The program has the potential to make you feel better still. Even women who are symptom-free can benefit from having more energy, greater

(continued on page 20)

The Body Blues Flow Chart

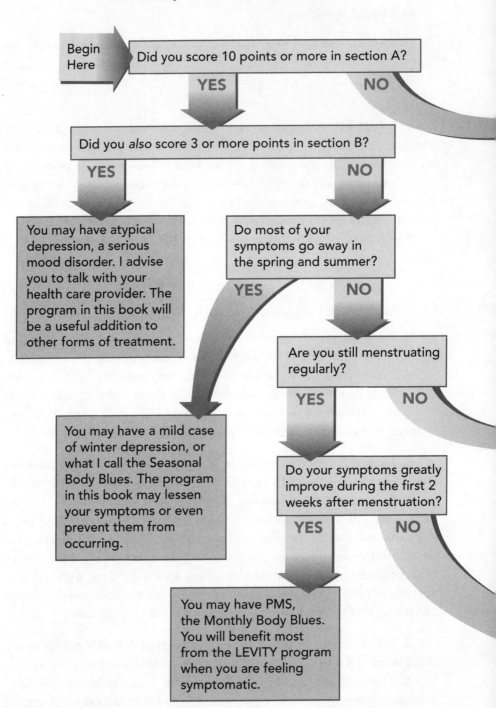

Begin Here

Did you score 10 points or more in section A?

YES   **NO**

Did you *also* score 3 or more points in section B?

YES   **NO**

You may have atypical depression, a serious mood disorder. I advise you to talk with your health care provider. The program in this book will be a useful addition to other forms of treatment.

Do most of your symptoms go away in the spring and summer?

YES   **NO**

Are you still menstruating regularly?

YES   **NO**

You may have a mild case of winter depression, or what I call the Seasonal Body Blues. The program in this book may lessen your symptoms or even prevent them from occurring.

Do your symptoms greatly improve during the first 2 weeks after menstruation?

YES   **NO**

You may have PMS, the Monthly Body Blues. You will benefit most from the LEVITY program when you are feeling symptomatic.

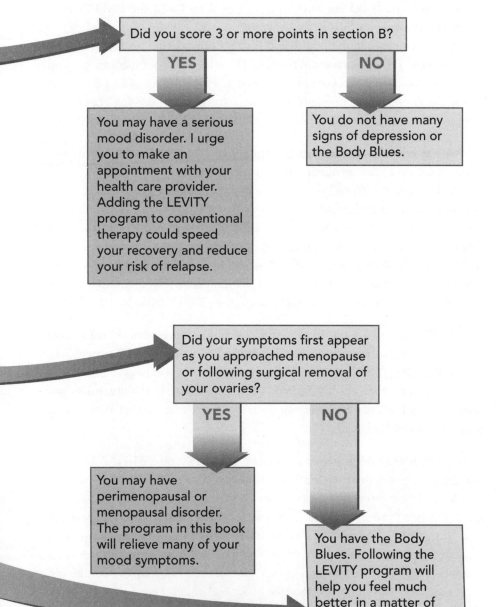

Did you score 3 or more points in section B?

YES

NO

You may have a serious mood disorder. I urge you to make an appointment with your health care provider. Adding the LEVITY program to conventional therapy could speed your recovery and reduce your risk of relapse.

You do not have many signs of depression or the Body Blues.

Did your symptoms first appear as you approached menopause or following surgical removal of your ovaries?

YES

NO

You may have perimenopausal or menopausal disorder. The program in this book will relieve many of your mood symptoms.

You have the Body Blues. Following the LEVITY program will help you feel much better in a matter of weeks.

immunity to stress, and another tool to help them maintain a healthy weight. In addition, taking part in the program could also reduce your risk of a number of serious health problems, including cardiovascular disease, diabetes, and cancer—a benefit I'll be discussing later on.

Q. I'm already taking antidepressants. Can I add the LEVITY program to my prescription drug therapy?

A. Yes, you can. In fact, there is growing evidence that each of the three components of the program will enhance the effects of your medication. You are likely to experience greater symptom relief and may even be able to lower the dose or transition off the drug. Before you make any changes in your medication, of course, seek the advice of your health care practitioner.

Q. I'm a health professional, and I'd like to learn more about the science behind your program. How can I do that?

A. We have referenced many of the key findings discussed in this book. You will find the notes on page 193. Also, you can read the paper that summarizes our results. We have reprinted the article with permission on page 172 of this book. Finally, we invite you to visit our Web site www.thebodyblues.com and click on the "News" section. This is where we post new findings about vegetative symptoms of depression and the proven benefits of bright light, moderate-intensity exercise, and the nutrients in the LEVITY formula.

Q. My problems seem to be due to perimenopause. Would it be wise for me to add hormone replacement therapy to the LEVITY program?

A. It is likely that increasing your estrogen levels will help relieve some of your vegetative symptoms. But you need to be aware of the potential consequences of hormone replacement therapy. Please discuss this matter with your primary care provider.

Q. I think my Body Blues is entirely due to stress. Will the LEVITY program help me deal with all the pressure I'm under?

A. Moderate-intensity exercise, one of the main components of the program, has been proven to relieve anxiety and help keep a stressful situation from turning into depression. I have relied on exercise to manage my own stress and anxiety for at least 25 years. Some of the ingredients in the LEVITY formula are also proven stress relievers. One of the most frequent comments from our study participants is that the program helped them cope with pressure. Also, consider counseling as a way to address the underlying causes of your stress.

Q. At various times in my life, I've had PMS, SAD, and peri-menopausal symptoms. Is this possible?

A. It's not only possible, it's common. Having one condition characterized by the Body Blues increases the likelihood that you will have the same cluster of symptoms at other times of your life. For example, a woman with PMS is more likely to have postpartum depression and experience a more difficult transition through menopause than a woman without PMS.

Q. I think my whole family has the Body Blues. Can my children take part in the program, too?

A. Brisk walking is beneficial for people of all ages. Your children will also benefit from getting more natural light. When children get too little light and exercise, they are more likely to feel grumpy and irritable, eat too much, and gain weight. They, too, get the Body Blues. The disorder is especially common in adolescent girls. Before you give them the vitamins and minerals in the LEVITY supplement, however, check with your primary care provider.

Q. I'm a guy, but I happened to take this test. I scored 25 points in section A. Do I have the Body Blues? Will the LEVITY program work for me?

A. You may indeed have the Body Blues. Although women are more likely than men to have vegetative symptoms of depression, men get them, too, especially after the age of 45 or 50. Will the program work for you? We did not test the program on men, so we cannot say yes unequivocally. However, all of the individual components of the program—light, exercise, and vitamins and minerals—have been shown by other investigators to improve men's moods. I recommend that you give it a try.

Chapter 2

The Biology of the Body Blues

Why Women Are at Greater Risk Than Men

In my work at the University of Washington Women's Health Care Clinic, I've discovered that the more a woman understands the biology of the Body Blues, the less she blames herself for her symptoms. Without this knowledge, many of my patients think that their symptoms are caused by a lack of willpower, laziness, or, as the Victorians called it, "sheer cussedness." This is rarely the case. In the last 10 years, scientists have learned that every symptom of the Body Blues can be traced back to some aspect of a woman's physiology. Of course, there are many other factors that influence a woman's risk of having this syndrome, including her upbringing, lifestyle, relationships, social status, and external stresses. But, as you will see, a woman's gender-specific biology plays a significant role.

In this chapter, you'll learn how three key hormones—estrogen, progesterone, and testosterone—influence the Body Blues. As you will see, your hormones fluctuate wildly throughout the month and throughout your life span. When certain hormones are at low ebb, you are most likely to have vegetative depressive symptoms. Although the LEVITY program will not alter your hormone levels, it *will* relieve the overeating, low energy, irritability, and foggy thinking that can accompany the fluctuations.

Estrogen: The Energetic Hormone

The best way to understand the mood and mental effects of estrogen, progesterone, and testosterone is to see how they interact over one menstrual cycle. What you learn about these hormones will have relevance to you whether you are having regular periods or have already gone through

menopause. Adult women of all ages have the same hormones, just in dif-
fering amounts.

The graph below shows how estrogen levels change across a typical
menstrual cycle. As you can see, the monthly rise and fall of estrogen looks
like a roller-coaster ride with two hills, the first one steeper than the second.
(Note: This graph focuses on estradiol, one of three compounds that are
known collectively as estrogens.)

Estrogen rises from the lowest to the highest level during the first 2 weeks
of the cycle. As a result of this abrupt rise in estrogen, an egg begins to ma-
ture in the follicles, a fact you may recall from a high school health class.
Research conducted in the past 10 years has revealed that this same monthly
surge influences virtually every aspect of a woman's being, including her
supply of serotonin. Researchers are discovering that estrogen enhances serotonin activity in multiple ways. The hormone appears to (1) create more receptors to grab on to serotonin, (2) prevent serotonin from being taken out of
circulation, and (3) speed its production.[1] Greater serotonin activity is linked
with a better mood, reduced appetite, more physical energy, and more resilience to stress. Serotonin is a potent antidote to the Body Blues.

Estradiol Levels over One Menstrual Cycle

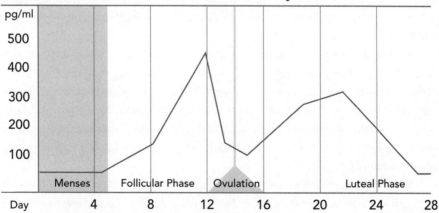

*This graph shows typical estradiol levels (measured in picograms per milliliter) over
one menstrual cycle. The gray bar represents 5 days of menstruation, and the gray
triangle indicates the day of ovulation. Estradiol rises to a peak just before ovulation, declines during ovulation, then rises to a lower and broader peak in the
second half of the menstrual cycle.*

In addition, estrogen may increase the brain's supply of dopamine,[2] which is the main player in the body's "reward system." Dopamine is the chemical that is released when you take part in fundamental and enjoyable activities such as eating and having sex. To give you some idea of dopamine's seductive power, it is the very same chemical that is triggered by using illegal street drugs such as cocaine or methamphetamine.

Meanwhile, estrogen is having another potent effect on your mind by increasing the amount of blood that flows to your brain.[3] It does so by relaxing key arteries, allowing more blood to pass through. When cerebral blood flow is high, people have a better memory, perform better on tests of verbal fluency, and are less likely to be depressed.[4]

A new finding that has stunned researchers is that a woman's monthly rise in estrogen also makes her brain cells more "connected" for the first 2 weeks of the cycle.[5] In the past, the scientific community believed that the brain changed very little in adulthood, except to wither with age. Now there is growing evidence that estrogen stimulates the creation of a more extensive neural network.[6] The more neural connections you have, the better your brain functions. You talk more quickly, choose the intended word more accurately, find it easier to recall names, spell better, and think more quickly.[7] One team of investigators found that young women do better on certain memory and cognition tests during the first phase of their menstrual cycle, which is when estrogen may be giving them a richer network of neurons.[8] One might liken estrogen to Miracle-Gro for the brain.

Estrogen is an energy booster as well. The word *estrogen* comes from the Latin word *oestrus*, meaning "frenzy." When animals are ovulating, they become very active, which is why this period of the reproductive cycle became known long ago as the estrus. When scientists isolated the hormone that is responsible for all this frenzy, they named it "estrogen," or the hormone that produces estrus. For women, too, a high level of estrogen is linked with more physical energy.[9]

When you combine all of the benefits of rising estrogen levels, you can begin to see why many women feel best during the first half of the menstrual cycle. The surge of estrogen is giving them a brighter outlook on life, taming their appetites, improving their memories, helping them think more clearly, and giving them more energy. As one of our LEVITY volunteers said, "This is the time of the month when I start a new diet, join a gym, and do all the chores I've put off for weeks. I even floss my teeth every day."

The Fall

Now take a moment to look back at the graph "Estradiol Levels over One Menstrual Cycle" on page 23, and you will see that estrogen starts to decline just before ovulation. As estrogen production slows, it appears that (1) serotonin and dopamine become less available to the brain, (2) cerebral blood flow diminishes, and (3) the neural network begins to shrink. Given these facts, one would think that women would feel confused, moody, ravenous, and irritable after ovulation. In a minority of women, this is indeed the case. A significant number of women have a mild case of the Body Blues around the time of ovulation and may even gain a couple of pounds. But most women handle this first drop surprisingly well. Once estrogen hits bottom a few days after ovulation, it climbs upward again, although this time the incline is less steep. After this second rise, estrogen coasts back down to the bottom, and menstruation begins.

For reasons yet unknown, it is this second withdrawal of estrogen that can trigger the most mood problems. According to one theory, the first hormonal plunge sensitizes the body so that the second withdrawal has more impact. (This is referred to as the kindling effect.) Whatever the reason, as many as 70 percent of all women respond to this second fall of estrogen with mild to severe vegetative symptoms of depression. As the roller-coaster ride glides to a stop, sleep becomes more elusive to women, the chocolate ice cream disappears from their freezers, carbohydrates call out in the night, thinking becomes less focused, and every movement can seem to take a little more effort.

This Is Your Brain on Progesterone

Now let's take a moment to see how progesterone influences the Body Blues. The graph on page 26 shows estrogen and progesterone levels over one menstrual cycle. (Progesterone is represented by the dashed line.) As you can see, progesterone production is very low throughout the first half of the menstrual cycle, allowing estrogen to dominate. In the final 2 weeks of the cycle, progesterone starts to climb, eventually eclipsing estrogen.[10]

One of progesterone's most important roles is to support the implantation and growth of a fertilized egg. As is true for estrogen, however, progesterone influences your mind and mood as well.

Estradiol and Progesterone over the Menstrual Cycle

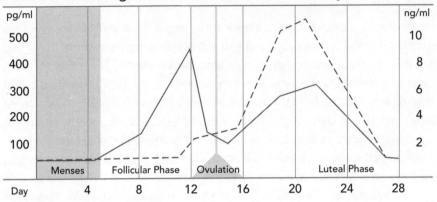

This graph shows levels of estradiol and progesterone (measured in nanograms per milliliter; see scale on the right) over the menstrual cycle. Progesterone is represented by the dashed line. Progesterone remains low until just prior to ovulation, then it peaks and eventually eclipses estradiol. Both progesterone and estradiol drop off sharply before the menses begins.

In general, progesterone seems to counter some of estrogen's actions, which is why some people refer to it as an *anti*-estrogen. A significant new finding is that high levels of progesterone may cause a slight *decrease* in the serotonin activity in the brain.[11] It may also slow cerebral blood flow.[12] Yet another discovery is that progesterone may prune back some of the neural connections that blossom when estrogen levels are high. (From animal studies, researchers have learned that progesterone can shrivel nerve connections in just 8 to 12 hours after administration.)[13]

Much research remains to be done in this area, however, including whether natural and synthetic forms of progesterone act in a similar manner. In general, the synthetic progesterones used in conventional hormone replacement therapy (HRT) appear to have more negative effects. And even though the body's natural production of progesterone may also cause a downturn in mood and mental functioning, the effects are relatively mild in most women. They are still able to perform all their normal functions.

Furthermore, progesterone, like estrogen, offers a number of benefits as well. It appears to enhance sleep, calm anxiety, and soothe irritability. Some people refer to estrogen as a natural antidepressant and to progesterone as a natural antianxiety compound. In a revealing experiment, researchers gave 400 milligrams of natural progesterone to a 55-year-old woman who had had her ovaries removed and was producing little of the hormone on her own. Within 30 minutes of taking the hormone, she felt very sleepy. At the end of an hour, she had lost her ability to concentrate and was talking incoherently. Then she fell sound asleep and could not be awakened for another hour. When she woke up, she could not remember anything beyond the first 30 minutes of the experiment.[14]

Partly because of the sedating properties of progesterone, some women experience a good mood in the first week after ovulation, which is when they have relatively high levels of both estrogen and progesterone. In this brief window of time, progesterone is tempering the activating effects of estrogen, which can result in a tranquil but alert state of mind.

> ## PMS: The Monthly Body Blues
>
> "WHEN MY PERIOD IS OVER, I usually feel great. Not just in one part of my life but all parts. I exercise more. Eat less. I'm more outgoing. I pay my bills on time. Clean up my office and take my clothes to the dry cleaners. And I can even lose 1 or 2 pounds. Then midcycle, the world seems to turn upside down. I feel tired. I wake up during the night and can't get back to sleep. Sometimes, I don't even feel like answering the phone or answering my e-mail. Every month, it's one step forward, one step back. I don't make any progress. I've been doing this for the past 15 years."
>
> **LEVITY volunteer, 43**

When progesterone falls off at the end of the cycle, women lose its tranquilizing, sleep-enhancing properties. Surveys show that women wake up more often and spend more time awake during the night in the days before their menses than at any other time of the cycle.[15] Some maintain that the withdrawal of progesterone may also add to the irritability and mild anxiety that some women experience in the days before menstruation.

This Is Your Sex Drive on Testosterone

The final hormone in the monthly trio is testosterone. Many people are unaware that women produce testosterone. Indeed they do, although men have 14 to 18 times more, justifying its designation as "the male hormone." In years past, people thought that estrogen was the driving force behind women's sexuality because it peaks just prior to ovulation. It also keeps the vagina moist and supple, facilitating intercourse. But it now appears that estrogen has little influence on women's desire for sex or their physical sensations.[16] Testosterone is the hormone that fuels their desire and enhances their pleasure, just as it does in men. When a woman has relatively high testosterone levels, she is more likely to think about sex, masturbate, respond to a partner's advances, and initiate sex. When she has low testosterone levels, she is more likely to say no to her partner and be less interested in all types of sexual activity.[17]

Barbara Sherwin, Ph.D., professor of psychology at McGill University in Montreal, has taught us a great deal about women and testosterone. Dr. Sherwin is a psychoneuroendocrinologist, a specialist with expertise in three related fields of study: psychology (the mind), neurology (the nervous system), and endocrinology (the hormonal system). These qualifications make her supremely qualified to untangle the complex link between our moods, brain chemicals, and hormones. She began her research in the early 1980s as part of an investigation of women who had had their ovaries removed. (A woman who has gone through surgical menopause is an ideal candidate for hormone research because she has low levels of all the reproductive hormones. A researcher can give her individual hormones and study the effects of each one in isolation.) Dr. Sherwin found that giving testosterone to the women increased their desire for sex, gave them more pleasure during intercourse, and even intensified their orgasms. Women who had gone through natural menopause responded in a similar fashion when given testosterone.[18]

Since those early studies, other researchers have found that supplemental testosterone can boost the sex drive of healthy younger women as well.[19] In one study, eight women with functional ovaries and a healthy interest in sex were given testosterone supplements. Within 4 hours, the extra helping of testosterone increased their "genital sensations" and feelings of "sexual lust."[20]

Testosterone may give women other benefits as well. In one study, Dr. Sherwin gave estrogen alone or estrogen along with a low dose of testosterone to a group of women who had undergone surgical menopause. The women given the testosterone felt more composed, elated, and energetic than those given just the estrogen.[21] From these and other studies, it appears that testosterone may be a four-in-one tonic for women: It can enhance their sexuality, relieve their fatigue, improve their mood, and calm their anxiety.

As is true for estrogen and progesterone, however, testosterone also varies across the menstrual cycle. It is low during the first part of the cycle, peaks at ovulation (good planning), and then declines during the final 2 weeks. You can see this gentle rise and fall on the graph "One Woman's Mood Map of the Menstrual Cycle" on page 30. (Testosterone is represented by the dotted line.) Besides these monthly ups and downs, women also produce lower amounts of the hormone as they age. A typical 40-year-old woman may have half the amount she did at age 20.[22] She also lacks the midcycle surge of the hormone, which can eliminate the monthly peak in sexual desire she experienced in her youth. There is growing evidence that at least some vegetative symptoms of depression—especially fatigue, anxiety, and low sexual desire—may be due, in part, to a woman's variable supply of testosterone.

In addition to the natural cycling of her hormones, there is another time when a woman can have low testosterone levels—when she takes supplemental estrogen, whether in an oral contraceptive or a hormone replacement therapy regimen. In a current study, postmenopausal women who were given a daily dose of 2 milligrams of natural estrogen (oral micronized estrogen) registered a 42 percent *decrease* in their testosterone levels.[23] In recent years, a number of HRT preparations that include testosterone have appeared on the market. However, many health care practitioners, myself included, are waiting for further evidence that long-term testosterone use in women is free of unwanted side effects. Larger studies are now underway.

The Best and Worst of Times

Now that you have this brief overview of the three reproductive hormones, it's time to look at their combined influence on women's moods. Take another look at the graph "One Woman's Mood Map of the Menstrual Cycle" on the following page. As you can see, estrogen is represented by the smooth line, progesterone by the dashed line, and testosterone by the dotted line.

Directly below the graph is a segmented bar that illustrates how a woman might feel at the various stages of her menstrual cycle. The white segment on the band represents the time when she has the fewest symptoms of the Body Blues. As you can see, this is the part of the cycle when she has rising estrogen and testosterone levels but minimal progesterone. For her, this is the ideal mix of hormones. Together, the two energizing hormones increase her energy level, enhance her mood, clear her thinking, spark her sexual desire, and reduce her appetite.

The light gray segments on either side of the white segment mark those times when she has relatively few mood problems but does not feel quite as energized or high-spirited as she does when her estrogen and testosterone levels are higher.

The two dark gray segments on the ends of the bar indicate those times when she is most likely to be troubled by food cravings, weight gain, fatigue, and mood swings. This high-risk zone includes the 4 days on either side of the first day of menstruation—8 or 9 days in all. Over this stretch, she has low levels of all three hormones—the monthly ebb tide. She lacks the energizing effects of estrogen and testosterone and the calming effects of progesterone. There is an un-

One Woman's Mood Map of the Menstrual Cycle

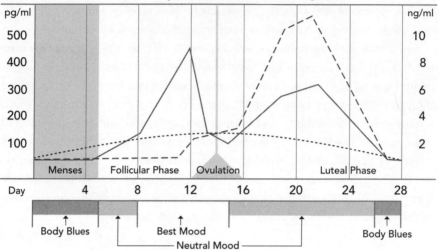

This graph illustrates the levels of estradiol, progesterone, and testosterone (dotted line) over one menstrual cycle. Testosterone (measured in nanograms per milliliter) has a slight rise from the time of menses to ovulation, then a gentle decline back to low levels.

The shaded bar below the graph is an example of how a particular woman might feel during parts of this complex hormonal cycle. Each woman's mood map is unique. The darkest segments represent those times when she has symptoms of the Body Blues, including fatigue, irritability, sleep difficulties, and low-level anxiety. The light gray segments indicate times of the month when she has relatively few symptoms. The white segment prior to ovulation represents the time of month that she has the fewest symptoms and the best mood.

wieldy term for this part of the menstrual cycle—the *perimenstrum*, which means "the time surrounding menstruation." (It differs from the *premenstrual* part of the cycle in that it also includes the first days of menstruation.)

I want to emphasize that each woman's menstrual mood map is unique. Some women have a low mood as soon as they reach ovulation and continue to feel moody until they are through menstruating. Some women have premenstrual symptoms twice a month—once right after ovulation and then once again during the last 5 or 6 days of the cycle. Altogether, four common variations of PMS have been identified. Some lucky women, about 30 percent of women in their reproductive years, escape the monthly Body Blues entirely.

Also, it's important to note that no matter what blend of hormones a woman happens to be "on" at any given time of the month, life events can easily override their influence. If something tragic happens to you when your estrogen is on the rise, for example, you will still experience grief and sorrow. You can even feel very depressed. Or if something wonderful happens to you just before menstruation, you can forget all about the premenstrual blues.

But if you stand back far enough and look at all American women between the ages of 11 and 50, one part of the menstrual cycle stands out from all the others—the days just before and after the first day of menstruation. Surveys show that women who are in this part of the cycle are more likely to be admitted to hospitals for psychiatric reasons,[24] have episodes of bingeing,[25] attempt suicide,[26] have migraine attacks, commit violent crimes,[27] consume more calories, feel anxious, and have episodes of acute panic.[28] Clearly, the monthly rise and fall of hormones can have a significant impact on women's well-being.

Pregnancy, Nursing, Perimenopause, and Menopause

How do the new discoveries about hormones and mood apply to women who are *not* having regular menstrual cycles? When women are pregnant, breastfeeding, or menopausal, both the monthly hormone swings *and* the accompanying mood swings are greatly diminished. The same three hormones are still present, however, and they still have considerable influence on how a woman feels and functions.

To explain how hormones influence women's moods across their entire life span, not just one menstrual cycle, would require several books, not just a part of one chapter. But a lot can be learned simply by looking at one hormone—estrogen—and seeing how it varies across a typical woman's life span. As you look at the graph on page 32, keep in mind that every time there is a dip in the level of estrogen, a woman may be experiencing a reduction in the dopamine and serotonin activity in her brain, less blood flow to her brain, and a decrease in the interconnectedness of her brain cells.

Each of the shorter, jagged peaks on the graph represents the rise and fall of estrogen over one menstrual cycle. (The area under the magnifying glass gives a close-up view of one cycle.) This monthly ebb and flow begins when a girl menstruates for the first time, typically between the ages of 11 and 14. National statistics show that this is also the first time that females begin to have more mood problems than males do.[29]

When a girl starts to menstruate, both her cycles and her mood can be erratic. As she matures, she begins to experience a more rhythmic surge and withdrawal of estrogen every month. This is also when she can begin to have monthly bouts of the Body Blues. Symptoms of PMS are most common in women between the ages of 20 and 40.

Estrogen Levels over a Woman's Life Span

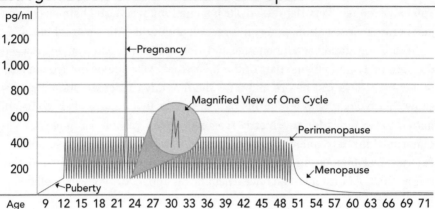

This graph gives you a rough idea of changes in estrogen production over a woman's life span. Each of the short, jagged peaks represents estrogen production over one menstrual cycle. (As you can see in the expanded view, each of the lines should have a double peak of estradiol, as was shown in the previous illustrations of the menstrual cycle.)

The one sharp spike toward the left of the graph represents the tremendous increase in estrogen production over the course of one pregnancy. The spike could not be drawn to scale, because estrogen levels can increase one hundredfold by the third trimester of pregnancy. In reality, the spike should be about 30 times taller than the one shown here.

The tall single peak represents the rise and fall of estrogen over the course of one pregnancy. In the third trimester of pregnancy, estrogen levels can soar 100 times higher than during a typical menstrual cycle. Amazingly, within just 48 hours after giving birth, a woman's estrogen production comes crashing back to earth, returning to the levels that occur during a typical menstrual cycle. (Much of the estrogen was being produced by the placenta.) This hormonal riptide triggers a mild case of the baby blues in 50 to 80 percent of all new mothers.[30] The most common symptoms are mild depression, crying, irritability, anxiety, and fatigue. Fortunately, these symptoms disappear in a matter of days or weeks, demonstrating the resilience of the human body.

When and if a woman chooses to breastfeed her infant, her estrogen levels may sink even further and then stay low until the baby begins to get other forms of nourishment. (Frequent suckling suppresses ovulation and keeps estrogen relatively low.) Breastfeeding suppresses testosterone production as well, serving as a natural form of birth control.

On the right of the graph, you see estrogen levels during perimenopause. In the years leading up to menopause, a woman's menstrual cycles become more and more erratic. Starting in her middle thirties through her late forties, she begins to have changes in menstrual flow or the length of her menses. Then, in her midforties, she is likely to have changes in cycle length as well. In the end of the perimenopausal transition, she may start to skip periods.[31] Given the unpredictable nature of her hormone production, it's not surprising that she is at greater risk of having the Body Blues. Several studies have shown that women have more depressive symptoms between the ages of 40 and 50 than they do at any other time of their lives.[32,33] At the present time, approximately 20 million American women are weathering this rocky transition.

Finally, when a woman reaches menopause, her estrogen production drops sharply and then declines slowly for the rest of her life—unless she chooses to go on hormone replacement therapy. Some older women produce such small amounts of estrogen that it cannot be detected.[34] Despite the fact that older women have low estrogen levels, some of them feel remarkably well after menopause. It seems to be the *cycling* of hormones—not their absolute amount—that has the most effect on women's moods. Once women reach menopause, they can breathe a sigh of relief because they have finally stepped off the hormonal roller coaster. Premenstrual symptoms, the baby blues, and the perimenopause are all behind them. According to a British study, once women reach menopause, they are less excitable, irritable, and depressed.[35]

Even though postmenopausal women may have fewer mood swings, they still have to contend with very low estrogen levels and their well-known physical effects— hot flashes, urinary incontinence, vaginal dryness, and osteoporosis. In addition, low estrogen levels may decrease their cerebral blood flow and impoverish their neuronal connections, increasing the risk of

Postpartum Depression

About 1 out of every 10 women experiences more than a bout of the Body Blues after giving birth. She has a more serious reaction called postpartum depression, which requires treatment. On the extreme end of the spectrum, 1 out of every 1,000 women has a very severe reaction to giving birth called postpartum psychosis. This disorder requires immediate medical attention.

having problems with cognition and memory, and perhaps even Alzheimer's disease. Also, as women reach their seventies and eighties and begin to experience some of the inevitable losses of those later years, they have an increased risk of depression.[36]

Why Do Some Women Escape the Body Blues?

When you think about all of the times in a woman's life when she has low or fluctuating levels of estrogen, it seems as though all women should have the Body Blues at least some of the time. Why are a majority of women free of this syndrome? The answer is not yet known, but there are some intriguing clues, having to do with both genes and lifestyle.

One new finding is that the receptors for estrogen, serotonin, and dopamine come in several genetic varieties. Some women are born with receptors that are very good at holding on to these particular chemicals. During those times of their lives when they are producing less-than-optimum amounts of estrogen, serotonin, and dopamine, they can still utilize enough of the chemicals to sustain a good mood. Other women get a less fortuitous draw from the gene pool and have to cope with fewer or less efficient receptors. In the coming years, we will know a great deal more about these hidden genetic influences.

Another critical factor that influences whether or not a woman's normal cycling of hormones triggers the Body Blues is her lifestyle. As you will discover throughout this book, women who get regular physical activity, more exposure to natural daylight, and an adequate supply of certain key nutrients have many fewer problems with low mood, fatigue, stress, and overeating—even during those times of their lives when they have an "unfavorable mix" of hormones. The LEVITY program is designed to foster those activities and daily habits that have been proven to help eradicate the symptoms of the Body Blues. By making simple changes in your lifestyle that take no more than 20 minutes of your time, 5 days a week, you, too, can say goodbye to the Body Blues.

Men, Hormones, and Mood

Before I go into more detail about the LEVITY program, I want to take a brief look at men and their hormones. This glimpse from across the gender gap will give you a better perspective on some of the basic biochemical differences between men and women.

The primary reproductive hormone in men is testosterone. Like estrogen, testosterone can have a profound effect on mood. On the negative side, testosterone is linked with having more problems with anger and engaging in more risky, antisocial, and criminal behavior. But testosterone also gives men many advantages. Similar to the effects that estrogen has on women, testosterone stimulates serotonin activity,[37] boosts energy, and enhances mood. As an added bonus, it serves as a potent aphrodisiac.

Men also benefit from the fact that they produce a steady supply of testosterone from day to day and month to month. The graph on page 40 shows testosterone levels over a man's life span. As you can see, men produce high and steady amounts of testosterone throughout most of their adult years. There is no male equivalent to the rise and fall of hormones that women experience with each menstrual cycle. Nor is there anything that remotely resembles the cataclysmic rise and fall of estrogen that accompany childbirth. Most men enjoy a steady infusion of testosterone until they reach late middle age.

Men do not escape the Body Blues entirely, however. Around the ages of 45 to 50, they begin to experience a gradual but steady decline in testosterone production, a phenomenon that some people refer to as the *andropause*. In response to this gradual withdrawal of testosterone, some men experience a male version of the Body Blues. They have less energy, less sexual desire, more erection difficulties, less physical strength, more fatigue, and more memory problems. In addition, they have a greater risk of osteoporosis, insomnia, and weight gain, especially around the middle.[38] (One survey reported that men with low testosterone levels are also much more likely to "fall asleep after dinner.")

But in most men, these symptoms do not appear until they are over 40. In contrast, some women have to cope with the Body Blues starting with their very first months of menstruation. Also, a man's testosterone production decreases with age much more slowly than does a woman's estrogen production. For this reason, men's symptoms come on more gradually and are less disruptive.

Another little-known fact is that men produce a steady supply of estrogen as well as testosterone, although in small amounts (equivalent to what women produce in the first week or so of the menstrual cycle). Estrogen, like testosterone, is a unisex hormone. Men's production of estrogen does not fall off with age, however. As a result, many adult men have higher estrogen levels than menopausal women. (The normal range of estradiol in men is from 10 to 50 picograms per milliliter. Postmenopausal

(continued on page 40)

Using the Body Blues Symptom Log

On page 38, you will find a simple chart to help you keep track of the symptoms of the Body Blues. It will help you identify which symptoms are most troubling to you, when they occur, and which ones tend to be grouped together. This will help you understand your particular version of the syndrome. For example, without keeping a log, you may have the impression that you are feeling symptomatic much of the time. But when you take daily notes, you may see that your symptoms come and go and have a wide range of severity. Having this knowledge will help you predict when you are most likely to have symptoms and plan around them.

There's another benefit of keeping a log. Once you start the LEVITY program, your symptoms will become less bothersome. Because of your record keeping, you will be able to look back in time and see more clearly how the program has benefited you.

Directions: On the left-hand side of the chart, I have listed some of the most common symptoms of the Body Blues. (There are two blank rows at the bottom of the log for you to add additional symptoms.) Each day, look over the list and decide whether you've experienced any of the symptoms. If you have, rank their severity from 1 to 10, with 1 being barely noticeable and 10 being the most severe. (If you haven't been troubled by a particular symptom, enter a 0 or simply leave it blank.)

If you are having regular menstrual cycles, determine which day you are in your cycle, with Day 1 being the first day of menstruation, and enter your data in the column headed by that number. For example, if it has been 10 days since you started to menstruate, enter your data in the column headed by a 10. Each day, add up your total points in each column and write that number at the bottom.

If you are not having regular cycles, consider the numbers at the top of the columns as representing the days of the month, not the days of a menstrual cycle. If today is the 26th of the month, for example, enter your severity scores in the column headed by a 26. Then follow the instructions in the previous paragraph. Unlike a woman with regular cycles, you may not see a cyclical pattern to your symptoms, but you will see which ones are most troubling to you and how often they occur.

Make a special effort to enter your ratings on those days when you are having the most symptoms. These may be the very times when you don't want to add another chore to your already stressful day. But if you record your symptoms when you are feeling the most distressed, you will be able to identify your hormonal "hot spots."

The chart at the right is an example of one woman's mood ratings over a menstrual cycle. A couple of blank charts follow. (We give you permission to make copies of the blank charts so that you can keep a running record of your Body Blues. You can also visit our Web site (www.thebodyblues.com) and download additional copies.)

Example of a Completed Chart

Day	1	2	3	4	5	6	7	8	9	10	11	12	13	14	15	16	17	18	19	20	21	22	23	24	25	26	27	28	29	30	31
Symptom																															
Overeating	2	2	2	1	2	1	4	1	2	4	2	2	3	5	4	5	4	4	4	3	4	4	5	6	6	6	7	7	8		
Fatigue	3	3	2	1	1										2	3	2	3	3	4	5	7	7	4	6	5	8	8	8		
Tension	3	3	3	2	3				3			3	2			4	4	3			5	2	3	6	4	8	4	5	9		
Low mood	2	2	1	4	2	1	1	2	1	3	2	1	4	3	2	2	4	3	4	3	2	4	5	2	4	6	4	6	6		
Irritability	4	2	3	3	2	1	1	2	3	1	2	3	2		1	3	3	3	2	3	1	3	3	2	5	4	6	6	6		
Sleep problems	4	3	2	4	2	1	1	2	3	1	2	3	2		1	2	1	3	1	2	1	2	3	1	2	4	3	4	4		
Daytime drowsiness	4	2	3	4	3	4	5	4	5	4	5	6	4	5	3	4	5	4	5	6	3	4	5	3	5	4	6	4	7		
Low desire	1	1	3	2		2	2		1	2					2	1	2	5	3	6	4	5	3	5	1	1			1		
Feeling emotional	2	2	4	3	5		1	3			5	1		1	4	3	3	5				5	2	5	4	5	7	5	8		
Anxiety	1	2		1					1					1	2				1	2						2	3	3	4		
Sensitivity to criticism	3	2	2	1										1	2			2		1	1			3	2	4	4	4	6		
Forgetfulness					1											1						1									
Total	29	24	25	21	19	9	14	12	16	14	11	16	15	15	20	24	28	27	22	27	26	32	36	37	39	49	52	52	67		

(continued)

Body Blues Symptom Chart

Day / Symptom	1	2	3	4	5	6	7	8	9	10	11	12	13	14	15	16	17	18	19	20	21	22	23	24	25	26	27	28	29	30	31
Overeating																															
Fatigue																															
Tension																															
Low mood																															
Irritability																															
Sleep problems																															
Daytime drowsiness																															
Low desire																															
Feeling emotional																															
Anxiety																															
Sensitivity to criticism																															
Forgetfulness																															
Total																															

Body Blues Symptom Chart

Day	1	2	3	4	5	6	7	8	9	10	11	12	13	14	15	16	17	18	19	20	21	22	23	24	25	26	27	28	29	30	31
Symptom																															
Overeating																															
Fatigue																															
Tension																															
Low mood																															
Irritability																															
Sleep problems																															
Daytime drowsiness																															
Low desire																															
Feeling emotional																															
Anxiety																															
Sensitivity to criticism																															
Forgetfulness																															
Total																															

Changing Testosterone Levels over a Man's Life Span

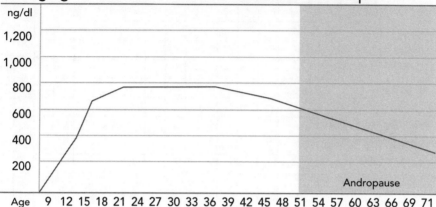

This graph shows typical testosterone levels (measured in nanograms per deciliter) over a man's life span. As you can see by looking back to the graph "Estrogen Levels over a Woman's Life Span," page 32, a man's testosterone production is much less volatile than a woman's estrogen production. Andropause can occur in the late forties or early fifties and continues as a man ages.

women have fewer than 15 picograms per milliliter.) In addition, men have a hidden supply of estrogen. Their brains contain large amounts of an enzyme (aromatase) that converts testosterone into estrogen. (The two hormones are both derived from cholesterol and have very similar chemical structures.) When you add up the amount of estrogen that older men have in their bloodstream plus the amount that they synthesize in their brains, they have *more* estrogen stimulating their neuronal network and cerebral blood flow than older women have.[39] This may be why women have twice the risk of Alzheimer's disease as men, even when women's greater life span is taken into account. Estrogen is a man's stealth weapon against dementia.

The LEVITY Program Evens the Score

If women produced their hormones in the same steady way as men, they would be less likely to have the Body Blues. For example, one way to prevent PMS is to take a drug that suppresses ovulation and smooths out the monthly hormonal peaks and valleys. When women have fewer hormonal swings, they have fewer mood swings as well. But whenever the normal cycling of women's reproductive hormones is stilled for whatever reason—birth control pills, anorexia, breastfeeding, strenuous athletic training, removal of the ovaries, or natural menopause—women cannot conceive. Hormonal swings go along with being the bearers of children.

One of the lessons that my colleagues and I learned from the LEVITY study, however, is that you do not have to alter your normal hormone production to get relief from the Body Blues. You can prevent your hormonal swings from becoming mood swings by taking part in the LEVITY program. When you energize your body through light, exercise, and vitamins, you lessen the fatigue, stress, and food cravings that are triggered by cycling hormones. What's more, these simple activities do more than relieve your symptoms; they also get at their underlying causes, including low activity of serotonin and dopamine and diminished blood flow to your brain. You will be learning more about these benefits in the chapters to come.

Chapter 3

The LEVITY Program

The Drug-Free Solution to the Body Blues

Just as quickly as the research community comes up with new insights into the biology of women's mood problems, the pharmaceutical companies rush to create new drugs based on those discoveries. They have given the highest priority to finding pharmaceutical solutions for women who feel tired and stressed and eat too much—products with tens of millions of potential customers. They've been making great strides. There are now designer drugs that can turn your appetite on or off, increase your energy, or give you a restful night's sleep with relatively few side effects. We are light years away from the Victorian remedies for the Body Blues of bloodletting and laudanum.

Despite the fact that the drugs are becoming more effective, many women don't want to take one pill to sleep, another to lose weight, and yet another to relieve stress and anxiety. They also worry about the high price of the medications. All in all, they would prefer a more natural solution. One person who became intrigued by the possibility of helping to create a drug-free treatment for the Body Blues is Jo Robinson, my coauthor. Jo is a best-selling freelance writer who specializes in mining the medical literature for overlooked studies that have great potential for improving people's lives. She began her latest quest several years ago with a deceptively simple question: "What makes women happy?" In particular, she wanted to find drug-free therapies that treated some of women's most common problems, including overeating, fatigue, and low-level depression.

Jo located a surprising number of alternative therapies that had been proven to relieve one or more of these conditions. Many of the therapies relied on aerobic exercise, while others focused on meditation, journal writing, light therapy, yoga, or specific vitamin regimens. But none of them had proven to be a comprehensive solution to the Body Blues. The therapies provided partial relief, treated only one or two symptoms, or helped a minority of women.

She wondered if combining several of the therapies into a single program might increase their effectiveness. She identified three promising activities that could be combined into a comprehensive therapy: (1) bright light, (2) brisk walking, and (3) a combination of six particular vitamins and minerals. But even though all three of these activities had been proven *individually* to relieve some aspect of the Body Blues, there was no guarantee that the three of them together would turn out to be an effective solution. To prove that the multifaceted program worked, it would have to be tested in a carefully controlled clinical trial.

Joining Forces

This is where I came in. Jo singled me out as a likely person to test her program idea because I was a researcher who had studied PMS and other women's issues. In addition, my training as a primary care nurse practitioner had made me very aware of the importance of educating my patients and helping them make positive lifestyle changes. (A nurse practitioner is a registered nurse with a graduate degree who is able to diagnose and treat illnesses and prescribe medications but has a special emphasis on counseling and health promotion.) Because of my background and training, I was just as interested in finding a practical application for my work as I was in doing the research itself.

When Jo explained the three-part program idea to me, I saw many points in its favor. It was simple and inexpensive, and it could be used by women from ages 18 to 80 and beyond. All told, it would take only 20 minutes a day. The program appealed to me for personal reasons as well. To begin with, light has always been very important to my sense of well-being. Throughout my adulthood, I've made a special effort to find apartments and houses with large windows, sometimes searching for weeks to find one within my budget. I have also lobbied for an office with windows, sometimes giving up other amenities just to be assured of getting enough light. I know from long experience that when I'm surrounded by natural light, I feel much better.

Exercise, another facet of the program, has been just as important to me. I started jogging when I was 30 years old and have included some type of exercise in my daily schedule ever since, even when I have been very busy. In fact, the busier I am, the more determined I am to squeeze in an exercise session because I know it will help manage my stress and anxiety. Now that I'm past 50, I appreciate the fact that exercise also reduces my risk of heart disease and cancer and strengthens my bones. But my main reason for exercising has always been to manage my mood and weight. Exercise calms me, energizes me, burns calories, and tames my appetite—a winning combination!

For these reasons, I enthusiastically accepted the challenge of developing and testing what would eventually become the LEVITY program. The study would be an excellent opportunity to add to the scientific understanding of the ways that light, exercise, and vitamins influence women's moods. More important, if the study yielded good results, it would offer a much-needed alternative for the tens of millions of women who are struggling with the Body Blues. They would no longer have to choose between drug therapy and no therapy.

Designing the Study

Within a few months of agreeing to test the program, I had assembled a research team, secured initial funding, and begun to design the actual study. My University of Washington colleagues and I decided that we would need to recruit about 100 women in order to have a valid study. Half of the women would take part in the LEVITY program itself, and the other half would be given placebos, which are sometimes referred to as "sugar pills." The reason for including a placebo group is that some people feel better simply because they *expect* to feel better, not because of any actual treatment.[1] For our study results to be accepted by the scientific community at large, the LEVITY program would have to be more effective than the power of positive thinking.

Once we were satisfied with our study design, we began recruiting volunteers. I was not looking forward to this part of the project. I knew from past experience that getting people to volunteer for a study can be a frustrating, time-consuming process. First of all, each participant has to meet a strict set of criteria; for every five people you recruit, perhaps only one will qualify. Then those who do qualify have to be willing to take part in the study even though they know they have a 50-50 chance of being assigned to the placebo group and getting only inactive pills. Understandably, some people drop out when they get this piece of news.

As part of the recruitment process, Jo and I arranged to be interviewed on a local talk show on KUOW, Seattle's National Public Radio (NPR) station. The interview was scheduled for the middle of July. As we were driving to the station, the sun was shining and there was not a cloud in the sky—a cause for celebration in "the Great NorthWet." But the sunshine only served to dampen *our* spirits because we worried that few listeners would be having mood problems on such a bright, sunny day. Would *anyone* volunteer for our study?

Fifteen minutes into the interview, the host of the talk show opened up the phone lines for questions. To our surprise, the switchboard lit up with calls from women wanting to know more about the Body Blues. "That's me you're talking about!" they said as if in one voice. For the first time, they had been given a name for their symptoms and a hope for a cure. When the host announced the phone number for people who wanted to volunteer for the study, the line became jammed with callers and stayed busy for the next 2 days. Some women told us they had to call more than five times to get an open line. From that one radio show alone, we recruited 463 volunteers—a response that was unprecedented in my 25 years of clinical research. It was suddenly clear to everyone on the team that the Body Blues was a major problem for a multitude of women.

Rainy-Day Blues

We scheduled the LEVITY study to begin in October, which is the beginning of the rainy season in Seattle. For the next 6 months, the Pacific Northwest would be blanketed in clouds. We chose this bleak time of year for a particular reason. Most people feel a bit down in the fall and winter, even those without winter depression. For example, a survey of 250 normal Boston women found that they had a drop-off in mood from August to January and then felt increasingly better from February to July.[2]

It was important that we avoid scheduling our study for a time of year when women would be feeling better spontaneously. If we did, critics could claim that the seasonal change, not the program itself, had caused the improved mood. By testing the program when our volunteers were on a downhill slide, we could show that any improvements were more likely to be due to the program itself. In fact, just keeping our volunteers on an even keel would be a noteworthy achievement.

The downside of starting the study in the fall was that it was going to make following the program more difficult for our volunteers. Walking outdoors in the late spring to early fall is a delight in our part of the world because the sun shines much of the time, the humidity is low, and the temperature rarely gets above 80°F. But in the late fall and winter, it's chilly and rainy much of the time. The women were going to have to put on their waterproof clothing and brave the elements when they would rather stay huddled indoors.

The decreasing hours of daylight would be another challenge. For the women to get maximum exposure to natural light, they would be walking outdoors during daylight hours. But in late November at our northern latitude (Seattle is at the same latitude as Quebec and St. John's, Newfoundland), the sun rises at 7:30 A.M. and sets by 4:30 P.M. Many of the women would be leaving for work in the dark and coming home in the dark for the duration of the study. In order to get in a daylight walk, they would have to find a way to squeeze an extra 20 minutes out of their workday.

On the positive side, the unfavorable weather and daylight conditions were going to be a worthy test of the program. In order for the LEVITY program to be a practical alternative to pharmaceutical drugs, it would have to be doable in all climates and at all times of the year. Women in Texas would have to cope with the summer heat, and women in northern Michigan would have to cope with the cold. If our Seattle volunteers were willing to walk outdoors when it was gray and raining, we would have a better idea whether women would follow the program during unfavorable weather conditions.

Launching LEVITY

Out of a total of almost 500 volunteers for the LEVITY study, 112 met all our criteria. (We excluded women who were too depressed or too happy, spent a lot of time outdoors, exercised three or more times a week, had physical problems that prevented them from walking, or took the same vitamins we were going to use in the study.) As we had hoped, the participants spanned the ages from 19 to 78 and included college students, single career women, full-time homemakers, working moms, and retirees.

To kick off the program, we invited the women to the University of Washington for an orientation session. When they arrived, they took five standardized tests.[3] Then we randomly assigned them to either the LEVITY program or the placebo group. (Of course, the women had no idea to which group they had been assigned.)

When the women assigned to the actual program arrived at their designated rooms, they learned about the three activities they would be doing for the next 2 months. Then they were given a supply of pills and a logbook to record their activities. We answered all their questions and then told them we would be seeing them again once the study was over. Unlike most studies that have explored the link between exercise and mood, we would not be supervising the women's walks or asking them to walk together in groups. The only support and monitoring they would receive was a biweekly phone call from a member of the research team. We designed the study to have minimal supervision because we wanted to see whether the women would complete the program if they received about the same amount of attention that they would get from a primary care provider. It was important to us that the program worked in the "real world," not just the laboratory.

Meanwhile, the women assigned to the placebo group were going through their own orientation. First, they watched a slide show about the nature of the Body Blues and the proven mood-enhancing effects of the vitamins and minerals in the LEVITY supplement. Then they were given a 2-month supply of pills. Unbeknownst to the women, the pills were made from inert ingredients that would have no effect on their mood. (To keep the identity of the pills a secret, the tablets were identical in appearance to the real vitamins.)[4] We told the women that a member of the research team would be calling them every 2 weeks to see how they were doing, which would be the same amount of attention given to the women taking part in the program activities. The women left the session with their placebo pills and a logbook to record their moods.

In academic circles, this group would be considered a very "active" placebo group. This means that we had given the women a number of reasons to feel better in addition to taking a pill. During the orientation session, we had helped the women feel more normal about their symptoms, given them new insight into the possible causes of their problems, and assured them that they would be getting a call from a member of the team every 2 weeks. It's been proven that simply giving people more attention can make them feel better, a phenomenon that has been referred to as the "Hawthorne effect." When the attention givers are trained healers, which was true in our study, the improvement is even greater. (All but one of our coaches were nurse practitioners.) Given these factors, it was likely that our placebo group would experience a noticeable improvement in mood.

The Results

For the next 2 months, the women in the placebo group dutifully took their pills and made notes in their logbooks. Meanwhile, the women in the LEVITY program took their pills, increased their exposure to light, went for frequent outdoor walks, and made notes in their logbooks. At times, the walkers were blessed with dry weather, but much of the time they had to slog through the rain. In fact, it rained 17 days during the last month of the program.

At the end of 8 weeks, it was time to see if the LEVITY program had relieved the Body Blues. All the planning, recruiting, screening, and coaching was finally over. We gave all the women the same mood tests that they had taken at the beginning of the study. When the results were compiled, we learned that both groups of women felt better at the end of the study than they had at the beginning. This is what we had anticipated. *But we were delighted to see that on every one of the five tests, the women taking part in the actual program had improved significantly more than those taking placebos, which is a rarity in clinical studies.* On one of the standardized tests, the LEVITY program had cut the women's depression scores in half. On another, the women as a group had moved from the worst to the best possible mood category.

Next, we took a closer look at the study results to see if the program had relieved the individual symptoms of the Body Blues. Once again, the program exceeded our expectations. As you can see in the graph below, the women who took part in the LEVITY program felt less stressed, irritable, anxious, and confused. They also had gained more control over their weight and appetite.[5] Furthermore, 25 percent of them had lost a noticeable amount of weight, even though we had not asked them to cut back on calories.

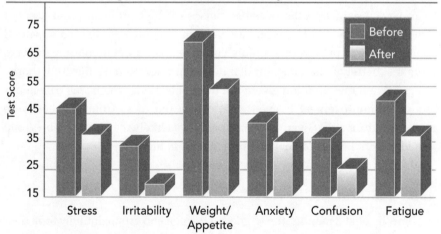

The LEVITY Program Relieves the Body Blues

This graph shows the before and after test scores of the women who took part in the LEVITY program. The dark bars represent the severity of their symptoms before taking part in the study, and the light bars show their scores once the study was over. The shorter the bars, the less the women were troubled by their symptoms. As you can see, the program helped relieve all six of these key symptoms of the Body Blues.

A More Intimate Look

In addition to reviewing the test results, we also interviewed each of the women who had been through the program. For me, this is one of the most rewarding parts of a study. Instead of studying data printouts and determining statistical significance, I get to see the impact my work has had on people's lives.

One of the women that I had followed throughout the study was a medical student who was at least 60 pounds overweight. When she was stressed, she would snack on sweets—and in medical school, the stress level is high much of the time. She would buy her favorite type of hard candy six bags at a time. Snacking and studying had become almost inseparable. "I would feel anxious whenever I was about to run out of the candy," she told me. "I'd even walk to the store late at night to buy more. I'd become addicted to this one type of candy, and nothing else would work."

Her reliance on the candy did not go away overnight. But after about a week on the program, she found that she was dipping into the bag less frequently. After another 2 weeks, she decided to see what would happen if she kept the candy out of sight. In its place, she put a bowl of grapes. It worked. "I'll still go for the candy when I am really stressed," she said, "but I no longer snack continuously." Gaining more control over her carbohydrate craving was already paying off. In 8 weeks, she had lost 5 pounds. "The funny thing is that I wasn't dieting," she said.

I also had a poignant interview with Rita, a 31-year-old single mother with a 12-year-old daughter. Before taking part in the study, Rita was feeling tired and low-spirited much of the time. She also had problems with low self-esteem. What bothered her most was that she and her daughter weren't getting along. "With just the two of us in the house," she said, "it can be very difficult."

About 3 weeks into the study, her daughter said to her, "Mom, you don't cry every day now." Rita had to stop and think. "I realized my daughter was right. My mood *was* better." During the last week of the study, Rita stepped on the scale and discovered that she had lost 4 pounds. "That's not much of a weight loss," she said, "but I never lose weight without dieting. It was actually kind of startling. I had to get off the scale and try it again."

She noticed other improvements as well. She was beginning to spend more time with an old friend. She had more energy for yard work. She painted her daughter's room, which was something she'd been promising to

We Can Change

> "I TOLD MY OLDER SISTER that I was taking part in the study. I told her I was having sleep problems, feeling tired, and eating too much. She said, 'Oh, we all have that! It's in the family!' Well, thanks for letting me know. But I found we can finally do something about it. We can make changes, and we can make ourselves better."
>
> **LEVITY volunteer, 33**

do for a year. Even her dreams had begun to change. "I used to dream about showing up for work naked. Or coming to work late and forgetting that I had an early appointment. Or I'd walk into a meeting, and everyone would be waiting for me. And there I'd be, naked." One night toward the end of study, she had a very different dream. "I dreamed that I showed up at work on time in a new suit," she told me. "Everyone told me how good I looked. I was on time for the meeting. Everything ran smoothly. I've never had that kind of dream about work before."

The members of our research team heard similar stories from the women they interviewed. An accountant who had felt severely stressed by her job before the study began said that she had improved so much that her coworkers wanted to know how they could take part in the program. A number of women remarked that their sex lives had improved. Said a mother of four, "Before, sex was not that interesting. But now, my husband and I are rediscovering each other." A woman who used to have great difficulty getting up in the morning said that she was now waking up before the alarm. "And I feel rested. It's like someone has shifted the hands on my body clock," she added.

The majority of the women told us they had more energy. They found their 20-minute walks had become easier to do. Some were going for longer walks, especially on the weekends. A few reported that they had started going for daylong hikes. Feeling better able to cope was another common refrain. One woman said, "I don't know if my life has become less stressful or if I'm just dealing with it better. But I'm taking control. Managing my schedule better. Prioritizing things."

Self-Empowerment Is the Key

Another theme that ran throughout the interviews was how much it meant to the women that they were getting better through their own efforts.

They reveled in the fact that it hadn't been a drug that had made them feel better; it had been their own effort and determination. One woman summarized the feelings of many others when she remarked, "The biggest benefit of the program was realizing that I can do it. I can do it! It's empowering to know that I have some measure of control over how I feel. I am not helpless. I am not without resources. I'm so glad I was listening to NPR that day and learned about the study. It's made a huge difference!" A second woman said it more succinctly: "I love knowing that I don't have to take any medicine to feel really great! I'm happy because of something I'm *doing*, not something I'm *taking*."

Since the completion of our study, we have learned that gaining a sense of empowerment over one's moods is one of the secrets to keeping the Body Blues at bay. Many people who have taken antidepressants are dismayed to learn that their symptoms return only a few months after they stop taking the drugs. Some people have to stay on the drugs permanently to keep from eating too much or feeling tired and irritable.

The relapse rate is much lower when people improve their symptoms through their own efforts. In a study at Duke University Medical Center in Durham, North Carolina, James Blumenthal, Ph.D., professor of medical psychology, and his team compared antidepressants with exercise. They found that 38 percent of the patients who had been successfully treated with antidepressants had sunk back into depression only 6 months after the end of the study. By contrast, only 8 percent of those who had walked their way out of a bad mood had relapsed.[6] Dr. Blumenthal speculated that the exercisers felt more responsible for their own recovery, which gave them a sense of competence and mastery that helped them maintain their good mood.[7]

My experience with the LEVITY project has led me to the very same conclusion. When women beat the Body Blues through their own actions, they not only feel good, they feel good about themselves. "I did it!" "I can stick to an exercise program." "I know that if I ever feel blue again, I have my own way of feeling better. I won't have to run to my doctor for a prescription." This

20 Minutes
to a Better Mood

"THE PROGRAM WAS A REAL eye-opener for me. Just this little bit of time. Really, I mean, really—just 20 minutes! It's not very long. But if you're doing the right things, it doesn't take much time to lift yourself up and begin to feel really good."

LEVITY volunteer, 42

feeling of self-confidence spills over into other areas of their lives, giving them more pleasure in the moment and more optimism about the future.

The women also regain mastery over their eating. As their tension and appetite begin to diminish, they find it easier to leave food on their plates, order modest meals at restaurants, and say no to dessert. Sweets and comfort food begin to take a backseat to healthy food. When they make better food choices, they enjoy their meals all the more. Their natural pleasure in eating is not undermined by feelings of guilt and self-criticism.

Ultimately, women discover that making a sustained effort to get more light, exercise, and essential nutrients has brought them closer to the healthy, happy lifestyle they have always envisioned. A 40-year-old LEVITY volunteer remarked, "The program was just what I needed to start turning my life around. Now I have a 3-year plan of how it's going to change. You know, I plan to live my life the way I'd like to live it!"

The fact that such a simple program could result in such a remarkable change is a cause for celebration.

PART 2

The Science behind the LEVITY Program

Chapter 4

Lighten Up!

The Mood Benefits of Recharging Your Solar Batteries

In this second part of the book, I'll be explaining why a simple 20-minute program can greatly relieve your Body Blues. As you will see, getting more bright light, engaging in moderate-intensity exercise, and taking the right vitamins and minerals can actually *reverse* many of the physical changes brought about by low or fluctuating hormones. These three activities boost the serotonin and dopamine activity in your brain, increase your cerebral blood flow, and reduce your stress hormones. As a result, you feel more energetic, think more clearly, have a better mood, eat less, feel more relaxed, and cope better with stress. This chapter takes a closer look at the proven benefits of the first activity in the program: creating a more natural lighting environment.

Reverence for the Sun

Throughout recorded history, people have worshiped the sun. Every known culture has created a sun symbol, and, invariably, it has been used to convey positive ideas such as energy, life, happiness, wisdom, and good fortune. Morning sunlight has been especially prized. In many traditional societies, people faced their dwellings toward the east so they would be greeted each morning by the full force of the rising sun. Today, millions of people in Asian countries still go outside each morning to practice ancient exercise disciplines such as tai chi or yoga, giving them the benefits of both exercise and sunlight.

In the Western industrialized world, our language is full of positive allusions to light. We talk about having a sunny disposition. We refer to that spe-

Lethargics

"LETHARGICS ARE TO BE LAID in the light, and exposed to the rays of the sun for the disease is gloom."

Aretaeus, Greek physician, 2nd century A.D.

cial someone as the light of our lives. We want to walk on the sunny side of the street. People we love brighten our days. We tell our somber friends to lighten up. A person whose brain is working well is a bright person. When we gain profound insight, we become en-lightened. The happy symbol that first became popular in the 1970s is a yellow circle with a smiling face—a veritable man in the sun.

When we want to express the opposite concepts—death, evil, sickness, depression, mental slowness, or suffering—we turn to words that convey darkness and night. Depressed people are in a dark or gloomy mood. (The word *gloom* comes from the Middle English word *gloming*—for "twilight.") A person with limited intelligence is a *dim*wit. When we are unaware of something, we are in the dark. Villains have dark scowls on their faces. A black cloak is worn by witches, the Grim Reaper, and Darth Vader.

Associating sunlight with happiness and darkness with depression and confusion is more than a metaphor. Most of us know from direct experience that we tend to feel happier on a sunny day and sad or moodier on a cloudy day. We also feel better in the summer than in the winter, even if we don't have an official diagnosis of seasonal affective disorder (SAD).

We've Moved Indoors

Despite our awareness that light enhances our mood, most of us are living a light-deprived existence. As soon as we leave our homes in the morning, we duck into a car, bus, or train. When we arrive at work, we scurry inside. After work, we run a few errands and then hurry back home. We spend most of our evenings cocooning indoors—reading, studying, catching up on paperwork, watching TV, listening to music, or being "mouse potatoes," the slang term for those of us who've become addicted to our computers.

This is a radical departure from the light-filled existence of our ancestors. Eons ago, our earliest ancestors spent the majority of their time outdoors because their very survival depended on capturing wild game and gathering wild plants, nuts, tubers, and seeds. Even as recently as 100 years ago, most people in rural communities still spent much of their time outdoors. To get from place to place, our great-grandparents walked, rode horses, or traveled by ox cart or buggy. Children walked to school, and the whole family walked to church. It wasn't uncommon for women to have to walk miles to visit their nearest friends or relatives. Women hung their clothes to dry on outdoor clotheslines and spent hours each day tending their gardens and livestock.

Because people spent so much time outdoors, their bodies were in sync with the rising and setting sun. Minutes after sunrise, the sunlight sent a signal to their pineal glands to shut down the production of melatonin, the body's calming, sleep-inducing hormone. At the same time, the light stimulated the production of serotonin and a host of other energizing, mood-elevating hormones and chemicals.[1] As a result, their hearts beat faster, their metabolic rate increased, and their brains became more alert. Thanks to the bright light, they were not merely awake, their minds and bodies were primed for the start of a new day.

Today, we are denying ourselves the energizing, synchronizing effects of bright light. We are awakened by our alarm clocks, not the sun, and we go through our morning routines in our dimly lit apartments and houses. The difference between the amount of light available indoors and outdoors is far greater than most people realize. We consider a room well-lit if it's bright enough for reading or doing detailed work. But even a brightly lit room has only a fraction of the amount of light available outdoors.

A common measurement of light is the *lux*.[2] On a sunny summer day at noon, there may be more than 70,000 lux of light outdoors. On a cloudy day, there may still be as much as 5,000 lux. Once we step indoors, the light level plummets; it's as if we had walked into a dense forest. For example, I have a sunny office at the university with large corner windows. Nonetheless, I get only 400 lux of light when I'm sitting at my desk. Most offices have 200 lux or less, even when all the lights are turned on. Our homes are darker still. According to Daniel F. Kripke, M.D., director of the Circadian Pacemaker Laboratory at the University of California, San Diego: "Many living rooms have only 15 lux of light, and some people watch TV in rooms as dim as 1 lux, which is about the same as the light of the full moon."[3] In truth, *we*—not our Stone Age ancestors—are the cave people.

Outdoor Light versus Indoor Light

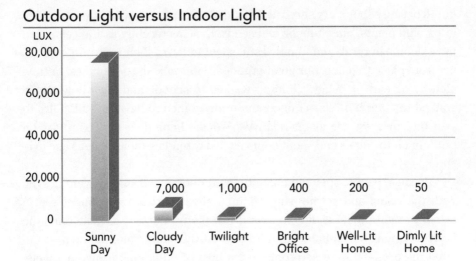

This graph shows the extreme contrast between the intensity of outdoor light and indoor light. The tallest bar shows the number of lux available to you outdoors on a sunny day. The next bar represents the amount of outdoor light on a typical cloudy day—100 times less than when the sun is shining. There is even less light at twilight. But the dimmest conditions of all are found indoors, as the next three bars illustrate. There is more than 1,000 times more light outdoors on a sunny day as in a dimly lit home.

Light and the Body Blues

A few years ago, Dr. Kripke and his colleagues decided to find out exactly how housebound and light-deprived we've become. The San Diego researchers randomly selected 150 middle-aged, middle-class adults and outfitted them with special wrist devices to record their light exposure 24 hours a day. The study began in August, a time of year when San Diego gets very little rainfall and the average daytime temperature is a delightful 74°F. Despite these idyllic conditions, half the people in the study spent less than 58 minutes a day outdoors.[4] The people who got the least light were outdoors for less than 13 minutes a day. Incredibly, for 12 hours of the day, the average light exposure was less than 100 lux.

Dr. Kripke and his team took the research one step further and decided to see if there was any link between the amount of time people spent indoors and their moods. *They found that the more time that their volunteers spent inside, the more tired, depressed, and anxious they felt, and the more they craved carbohydrates.*[5] By avoiding outdoor light, the volunteers had unwittingly turned summer into winter and given themselves a case of the winter blues. By contrast, those volunteers who spent more than 30 minutes a day outside had very few vegetative symptoms of depression. The natural daylight had energized their minds and bodies, helping them feel happy, active, and alert.

Why Women Need More Than Men

Although bright light is essential for the emotional well-being of both sexes, it may be even more important for women. As I explained in previous chapters, there are times throughout women's lives when they have less-than-ideal amounts of serotonin and dopamine, partly due to their fluctuating hormone levels. When women are deficient in these important chemicals, they are more likely to have the Body Blues. But, unwittingly, they increase their risk of feeling tired and stressed and eating too much whenever they spend most of their waking hours in a dim, indoor environment. Not only do they have to cope with their seesawing hormones, they are deprived of the stimulating effects of bright light as well.

Unfortunately, women are even more housebound than men. More women than men work at home, and as you have learned, homes tend to be more dimly lit than offices and factories. Those women who do work outside the home are much less likely to have outdoor jobs than their male counterparts. Also, women take part in fewer outdoor sports than men. It's not surprising that a later study conducted by the San Diego investigators found that women get significantly less light than men of similar ages.[6] This is the opposite of what should be happening. Because women have a greater risk than men of having the Body Blues, they should be getting more light than men do, not less.

Light Deprivation Depresses Mood More Than PMS

Surprisingly, in a British study, women's moods were more influenced by the amount of light in their environment than they were by their hormones. Dorothy Einon, Ph.D., a researcher from the psychology department of University College in London, designed a 1-month study to explore the connection between outdoor light levels and the moods of 39 college women.

During the study, the women kept daily mood diaries while the researchers kept careful track of the amount of light available outdoors. When the study was over and the women's moods were compared with the light measurements, the link between the two was obvious. As you might expect, whenever the sun was shining, the women as a group felt more cheerful. Whenever the clouds rolled in, the collective mood sagged. If a cloudy day abruptly followed a sunny day, the women's moods mirrored the change.[7] *What no one had anticipated, however, was that the light had a stronger influence on the women's moods than the phases of their menstrual cycles.* In other words, a stretch of cloudy weather could trigger a more noticeable dip in their moods than PMS.

The take-home message from these various studies is that it's not just fluctuating hormones that trigger the Body Blues—light deprivation can do so as well. As a result, you are more likely to have vegetative symptoms of depression during periods of cloudy weather, the short days of winter, and those times when you are in dimly lit indoor environments. For most women in our light-deprived culture, at least one or more of these factors are present virtually all of the time.

Impact of Light on Mood

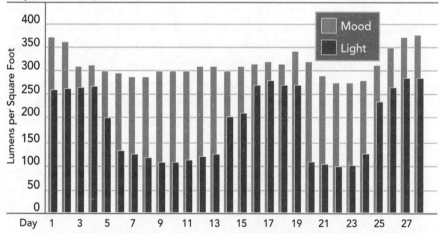

In this graph, the dark bars show how much light was available outdoors on each day. The higher the black bars, the brighter the light. The gray bars represent the women's average mood scores. The higher the gray bars, the better the women felt. As you can see, the women's moods went up and down along with changes in outdoor light. (Data from Einon 1997. Psychosom. Med. 59: 616–19.)

The Way to a Brighter Mood

These new findings about women and light raise an obvious question: If a lack of light increases your risk of having the Body Blues, will making a conscious effort to brighten your environment help relieve your symptoms? The answer is a resounding yes. In fact, you may feel noticeably better after spending just a few hours in a brighter environment.

To date, most of the evidence that light relieves vegetative symptoms of depression comes from studies of patients with seasonal affective disorder. In a typical experiment, the patients sit in front of a high-intensity artificial light source that emits from 2,000 to 10,000 lux of light. (Ten thousand lux is about the amount of light outdoors on a lightly overcast day.) The brighter the light, the less time the patients have to sit in front of the lights. In a few studies, blood samples have been taken before and after the treatment to measure changes in the patients' serotonin levels. The samples have shown that bright light stimulates serotonin activity in the brain, just as many anti-depressants do.[8] Within a few days, the patients have a better mood, eat fewer carbohydrates, feel more energetic, and become more outgoing.

Bright light may be even more effective in treating SAD than the widely

Bright Light Increases Serotonin

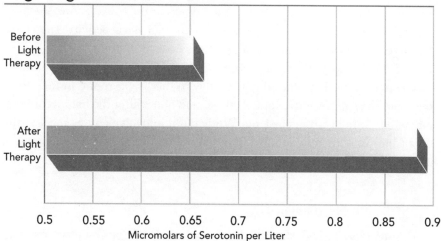

This graph shows blood levels of serotonin in people before and after bright light therapy. The bright light caused a significant increase in serotonin levels. Within a few days of treatment, the people experienced a brighter mood and had more energy. (Data from Rao et al. 1992. Acta. Psychiatr. Scand. 86: 127–32.)

prescribed antidepressant Prozac. In a landmark study, investigators compared the two therapies head-to-head. Light worked faster than the prescription medication, provided a greater degree of relief, and proved helpful for
twice as many patients.[9] When depression is due to a seasonal decline in daylight, bringing back the light may be the most logical *and* effective therapy.

But there is growing evidence that light therapy can relieve nonseasonal
depression as well. When it works, it does so very quickly. Antidepressants
can take from 2 to 3 weeks to kick in, which is a long time to wait if you're
feeling hopeless or suicidal. Bright light can improve mood in just a few days.
In fact, during the first week of therapy, bright light was proven to be three
times as effective as antidepressants.[10] Although light alone rarely brings
about full recovery from major depression, it is proving to be a valuable addition to more traditional therapies.

Light Equals Energy

By brightening your environment, you will be boosting your physical energy as well as your mood. No experiment demonstrated this more convinc-
ingly than a French study involving 13 healthy young men.[11] For a period of
a week, the men agreed to get up each morning and sit in a brightly lit room.
(The light in the room was about 2,000 lux. This is about 20 times more light
than found in a typical home, but less than what you would get outdoors
most days of the week.) After spending 2 hours in the bright room, the men
were given special wrist devices to measure their physical activity. Then they
were free to leave the lab and go about their normal routines.

The data from their wrist recorders showed that the men were much
more active when they started out the day in the bright room. In fact, they
continued to be more active until 9:00 P.M.—14 hours after the light treatment
had ended. Although this particular study did not involve any women, virtually all the phototherapy studies have shown that light has the same energizing effect on women.

Solving Sleep Problems

Getting more light during the day can also help you sleep better at night.
This is good news for the many women with sleep problems. According to
the 1998 Women and Sleep Poll conducted by the National Sleep Foundation,
sleep difficulties plague 71 percent of all women in the week before menstruation and 56 percent of all women in their perimenopausal years.[12]

Why does bright light help you sleep? When you get more light in the day-time, you produce more melatonin at night, which can result in a deeper sleep.[13] Bright light seems to be especially effective in solving the sleep problems of women 60 and older. In a 1993 study, older women who had more bright light during the daytime slept an extra hour each night. This was true for all of the volunteers, underscoring the effectiveness of the treatment.[14]

Light Up Your Mind

If you recall from chapter 2, when you have low or falling estrogen levels, less blood flows to your brain. Having low cerebral blood flow increases your risk of depression and compromises your ability to think. Getting more bright light has the opposite effect. Light stimulates your cerebral blood flow and helps relieve your low mood and confused thinking.

We owe this insight to a sophisticated technique called positron emission tomography, or PET, which measures blood flow to specific areas of the brain. Researchers have used PET scans to monitor the changes in cerebral blood flow in patients with SAD who are undergoing light therapy. Before light therapy, the scans show that the patients have reduced blood flow to the cerebral cortex, the "executive" part of the brain. Without adequate circulation, this critical part of the brain receives less glucose, its only energy source.

On the scans, this glucose deficiency shows up as a dark-colored area on the films. The darker the image, the deeper a person's depression. When depressed people say they feel "dim-witted," they are describing precisely the way their brains appear on a PET scan. After only a few days of phototherapy, however, this area of the brain begins to "light up," indicating greater activity. These phototherapy studies suggest that simply getting more bright light will increase the blood flow to your brain and relieve one of the hidden causes of the Body Blues.[15]

We Are Solar-Powered

Does sunlight have the same ability to relieve your vegetative symptoms of depression as artificial light? Until recently, it was impossible to say because virtually all the phototherapy studies used artificial light, not daylight. Now there is evidence that sunlight works just as well.

Anna Wirz-Justice, Ph.D., from the Center for Chronobiology at the Psychiatric University Clinic in Basel, Switzerland, decided to see if simply getting a group of patients with SAD to spend more time outdoors would help relieve their vegetative symptoms. For this pilot study, she recruited 20 patients (19 women and one man) and asked them to spend an extra hour a day outside. Although she did not ask them to exercise, most of the volunteers decided to use that time to go for a walk. After just 1 week of spending more time outdoors, the patients felt much better. In fact, taking a morning outdoor walk proved to be just as effective in relieving vegetative symptoms of depression as sitting passively for 2 hours in front of a light box.[16]

The Wirz-Justice study is one of the reasons that we decided to rely on natural daylight for our LEVITY program. We saw no reason to base the program on expensive lighting devices when daylight works just as well. Sunlight is free, and it's universally available. As the data from our own LEVITY study shows, there is even enough light outdoors on dark, rainy days to help women overcome the Body Blues.

Shedding New Light on Our Weight Problems

There is one key benefit of getting more bright light that has gotten very little media attention: Light alone can help you lose weight. In fact, this is one of the most consistent findings from phototherapy studies. After only a few days of bright light treatment, most people begin to eat fewer carbohydrate snacks—even if they are not trying to lose weight.

I want to take a moment to explore the close link between mood, light, and appetite, because overeating and weight gain are among the most common and troubling symptoms of the Body Blues. Studies show that the main reason that women overeat is that they are experiencing unpleasant feelings, especially anxiety, boredom, loneliness, fatigue, or sadness. Hunger motivates them only 10 to 20 percent of the time.[17]

When feeling distressed, most women prefer to snack on sweets and starches such as candy, cookies, bread, and baked goods. In one survey, 90 percent of the women but only 53 percent of the men said that they greatly preferred carbohydrate snacks over high-protein snacks such as cold cuts or cheese or salty snacks such as peanuts and pretzels.[18] Many women say that they prefer sweets because they like how they taste. But there is another, unconscious motivation for reaching for the doughnuts and cookies. Eating a carbohydrate snack boosts the serotonin activity in your brain, providing a short-term fix for the Body Blues.

Judith Wurtman, Ph.D., a research scientist in the department of brain

Why Do Sweets Boost Your Serotonin Levels?

Your body produces serotonin from an amino acid (protein fragment) called tryptophan. Tryptophan is abundant in various high-protein foods such as turkey, fish, meat, poultry, peanuts, cottage cheese, and sesame seeds. In order to be converted into serotonin, however, tryptophan must first enter your brain. The brain has a special barrier to keep out molecules such as tryptophan, so the amino acid has to be carried into the brain on a special transport mechanism. Think of this transport mechanism as a bus that carries passengers over a bridge.

Unfortunately, a lot of other amino acids want to ride on the same bus, and they outnumber tryptophan eight to one. In order for large amounts of tryptophan to enter the brain, the other amino acids have to be kicked off the bus. Paradoxically, the way to do this is to eat foods that are high in carbohydrates but *low* in protein. Eating sweet or starchy foods increases your blood sugar levels, which causes a surge in insulin. Insulin drives sugar out of the bloodstream, but it also clears the bloodstream of many of the competing amino acids. This leaves more room on the bus for tryptophan. Even though sweets contain very little tryptophan, there is enough of the amino acid in your body at any given time to take advantage of this free ride.

and cognitive sciences at the Massachusetts Institute of Technology, has conducted extensive investigations into the link between food and mood. In a 1989 study, she found that women with PMS who were given a single starchy meal experienced relief from virtually all of their symptoms in just 30 minutes. In particular, they felt less tense, angry, confused, and tired.[19] Her work suggests that eating that bag of chocolate chip cookies on the day before your period is more than an attempt to comfort yourself—it's an instinctual form of self-medication.

There are two obvious problems with the high-carb solution to the Body Blues. First of all, as little as an hour after eating a sweet or starchy snack, you have a noticeable dip in mood, so you have to eat more candy or carbs to keep feeling good. Second, you have to contend with all those empty calories. Dr. Wurtman found that women with PMS eat about 500 more calories per day in the last phase of the menstrual cycle compared with the first.[20] A woman who eats 500 extra calories for just 5 days out of the month can pack on an additional 10 pounds a year.

The Dopamine Fix

There's another hidden reason that women overeat: They may be trying to make up for a lack of dopamine. As I explained in chapter 2, the dopamine activity in your brain goes up and down with your estrogen production. When you have less estrogen, you have less dopamine activity. Your natural instinct is to find some way to replace it. Eating is one way to do so. Whenever you have food in your mouth, you have more dopamine activity in your brain.[21] This is nature's way of ensuring that people eat enough food to survive and reproduce. The fact that eating provides instant gratification makes us more willing to go to all the effort to bring in a steady supply of food.

Interestingly, food will give you a dopamine fix no matter what you eat. You can get more of this mood-enhancing chemical by eating a big bowl of fruit, a grilled steak, a tofu omelette, or a pint of Godiva Belgian Dark Chocolate ice cream. But the way to get the most dopamine is to eat food you really like, eat lots of it, and take a long time to eat it. The moment you stop putting food into your mouth, however, dopamine sinks back to its former level. *The only time that food gives you a dopamine high is when you are in the act of tasting, smelling, and chewing it.*

This phenomenon was demonstrated in a fascinating animal study published in 1996.[22] In this study, a group of rats was given a premeasured meal while the research team monitored the animals' dopamine production. As soon as the rats started to eat, the rodents had an instantaneous surge in dopamine. The level stayed up as long as the animals continued to nibble. But as soon as the food was gone, the dopamine surge vanished as well.

To learn more about this phenomenon, the research team gave another group of rats the very same premeasured meal. This time, however, they fed it to the rats in a tube that went directly into their stomachs. Although the animals got all the nourishment from the meal, they could not smell, taste, or chew it. Amazingly, with no sensory input, the rodents had no change in dopamine levels whatsoever; it was as if they hadn't eaten at all. In other experiments, scientists have blocked only the sense of smell of lab animals and have found that eliminating just this one sense gave the animals a smaller dopamine surge. The same appears true for us. In order to experience the greatest "high" from food, we need to be savoring its taste, texture, *and* aroma.

The fact that we humans produce more dopamine every time we put something tasty into our mouths may be the driving force behind the snack food industry. Perhaps the real reason it's impossible to "eat just one" is that one brief blip of dopamine is not enough. With each additional cookie, potato

Eating Increases Dopamine

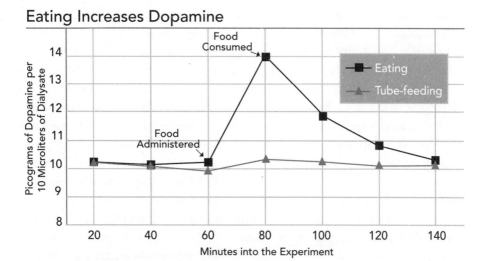

The peaked line marked with the squares shows the dopamine surge in rats that were able to smell, taste, and chew their food. The flat line marked with the triangles shows dopamine levels in rats that were deprived of sensory input and had the food injected directly into their stomachs. The study shows that the act of eating food stimulates an increase in the feel-good chemical. This appears to be true not only for rodents but also for humans. We need to savor food in order to experience more dopamine activity. (Data from Yang, Koseki, et al. 1996. Am. J. Physiol. 270 [2 Pt 2]: R315–8.)

chip, or piece of chocolate, we are prolonging the good feelings. If we snack on food that happens to be high in carbs and low in protein, which most women do, we are also stimulating our serotonin activity as well. It's no wonder that 90 percent of all women prefer carbohydrate snacks—nibbling on bread, pasta, and sweets can trigger two potent feel-good chemicals.

Unfortunately, as millions of women will attest, it's hard to sustain your good mood when self-medicating with food has made you gain weight and feel bulky, tired, and unattractive. Ultimately, overeating becomes a part of the problem, not the solution. Bright light is a far better way to relieve your symptoms. It not only boosts your mood, it also reduces your appetite, making it easier to lose weight.

Speeding Up Your Metabolism

Most of our understanding of light's ability to help people lose weight comes from studies of patients with SAD. People with SAD experience a strong carbohydrate craving and eat more food in the fall and winter than at any other time of the year. As a result, they can gain from 5 to 20 pounds each winter. When their mood rebounds in the spring, they spontaneously begin to eat less. But they still are burdened by their winter weight gain. Many people do not lose all the weight they gain each winter, so they add a few more pounds every year.

Getting bright light in the winter can prevent this seasonal buildup. In fact, one of the most reliable responses to light therapy is a decreased interest in food, especially carbohydrates. I'm pleased to report that sunlight has the same appetite-suppressing effect. In the Wirz-Justice study mentioned earlier, the women who went for daily outdoor walks began eating fewer carbohydrates in a matter of days. The effect was most noticeable in the second half of the day, which is when most women overeat.[23]

As an added bonus, there is some preliminary evidence that getting more bright light may also speed up your metabolism. In 2000, investigators at the Russian Academy of Medical Sciences used bright light therapy to treat a group of women with SAD.[24] To see if the light was having any effect on the women's metabolism, they monitored their oxygen consumption. (Oxygen consumption is a reliable indicator of metabolic rate.) The bright light did indeed increase the rate at which the women were burning calories. Even better, it helped them lose weight. By the end of just 1 week, the women had lost an average of almost 2½ pounds—an amazing amount of weight loss given the fact that they were not being required to diet or exercise.

New Hope for Obese Women

Bright light can even help the millions of women in this country who are significantly overweight. Many mysteries remain about why some people are so much heavier than others, but one new finding could be of some importance. In 2001, the journal *Lancet* published a study showing that the more people weigh, the fewer dopamine receptors they have in their brains.[25] (Receptors are structures that grab on to specific chemicals and make them available to the cells.)

People with clinically severe obesity have extremely low levels of the receptors. Even though they may be producing an adequate amount of dopamine, they can't utilize it well, which diminishes their sense of pleasure and well-being. This could be one of the reasons that they feel so compelled to eat. They have so little dopamine activity in their brains that they need to find some way to enhance it. Frequent eating is the most convenient way to do so. The more they eat, however, the more weight they gain, and the more despondent they feel about their inability to control their eating. These feelings of anguish can lead to yet more eating.

Bright light is one way to disrupt this downward spiral. In 1996, scientists enrolled four obese women in a 6-week pilot study. As in the Russian study just mentioned, the women were not asked to change their diets or exercise habits. All they had to do was sit in front of a moderate-intensity light box for 2 hours a day. (A brighter light would have shortened the exposure time to 30 minutes.) At the end of the study, three out of the four women had lost a significant amount of weight. They had also gained a better mood in the bargain.[26]

> ## Waking Up from Hibernation
>
> "LOOKING BACK AT MY HISTORY, when it was wintertime, I would pretty much hibernate, go inside the house, turn the blinds down, just kind of settle into the winter. Now I can't stand being in a dim room! I think the extra light has been a big factor in helping to curb my appetite. I've lost 5 pounds, which is wonderful, because I wasn't really on a diet."
>
> **LEVITY volunteer, 46**

In a similar experiment, researchers used bright light to treat 17 women with bulimia nervosa, an eating disorder sometimes referred to as "bingeing and purging." On average, the women had been struggling with bulimia for 12 long years. Each day for 3 weeks, the women spent 30 minutes a day in front of a 10,000-lux light box. Within days of starting the light therapy, they had fewer episodes of bingeing. When the women were switched to red lights (a color of light that does not alter mood or metabolism), they resumed their dysfunctional eating habits.[27] Light alone was able to disrupt a bingeing habit that was more than a decade old.

As you have seen, getting more bright light is a four-in-one diet aid. Light can (1) lift your spirits, which reduces your need to self-medicate with food; (2) increase your activity level, which helps you burn more calories; (3) suppress your appetite, which lowers your caloric intake; and (4) possibly even boost your metabolism.

Until modern times, women got all these benefits of bright light simply by going about their normal routines. Today, we have to consciously seek out the sun. All the billions of dollars that people spend on diet programs and low-fat or low-calorie foods might be better spent on skylights, sunrooms, outdoor recreation, and all-weather walking gear.

Bright Light in the Daytime, but Darkness at Night

When we coached LEVITY volunteers about the benefits of bright light, we also cautioned them about getting too much light at night. In order to defeat

Nighttime Ritual

"I'VE DEVELOPED a very pleasant night-time ritual. I get ready for bed by candlelight. There's something very soothing about it. Now when I turn on a bright light, I find it irritating."

LEVITY volunteer, 22

the Body Blues, you need to re-create nature's daily rhythm of light-ness and dark. Why is it important to turn down the lights in the late evening? Getting too much light at night can blunt your normal night-time rise of melatonin.

In a natural lighting environment, your body begins to produce melatonin at a regular time, typically around 9:00 or 10:00 P.M. (Adolescents and young adults tend to begin producing melatonin later at night, sometimes as late as 1:00 A.M. Older people may begin to produce melatonin as early as 8:00 P.M.) This nocturnal melatonin surge helps prepare you for sleep by lowering your heart rate, blood pressure, and body temperature. If you turn on bright lights at night, you blunt nature's Nytol, making it more difficult to wind down and settle into a deep and restorative sleep.

How much light is too much light at night? Less than you'd think. A decade ago, people thought that it took very bright light (5,000 lux or more) to interfere with the body's nighttime production of melatonin. Now we know that our bodies react very strongly to light in the first part of the night. From about 10:00 P.M. until 1:00 A.M., 100 lux of light is all that it takes to slow our melatonin production.[28] You can get this amount of light simply by being in a moderately well-lit room. If you customarily stay up until 11:00 P.M. or mid-night reading by the light of a 75-watt lightbulb, you are blunting your normal production of melatonin and could be robbing yourself of a good night's sleep.

In chapter 7, I will be describing some simple and inexpensive ways to create a more natural lighting environment. The more symptoms of the Body Blues you have, the more likely that you will benefit from making these changes.[29] What's more, you won't have to wait weeks or months to see re-sults. You are likely to feel better in just a few days. This healthy change in lifestyle has the potential to:

- Improve your mood
- Increase the circulation to your brain
- Boost your energy
- Curb your carbohydrate cravings
- Control your appetite in general
- Deepen your sleep

Chapter 5

The Walker's High
How Walking Beats the Body Blues

Y ou've probably heard of the "runner's high." This is the state of mind that allows people to smile as they run up steep hills, even though they are dripping with sweat. When athletes exercise at high intensity for 30 minutes or more, they produce endorphins, which are yet another class of natural substances that can create feelings of well-being.

But very few of our 112 study volunteers were able to exercise strenuously enough to experience an endorphin high. They didn't jog, work out at the gym, or even take regular walks. In other words, they fit the national norm. Today, only one out of four adults in the United States gets 30 minutes of moderate physical activity a day. Twenty-four percent have no leisure time physical activity whatsoever.[1] Women as a group are even more sedentary than men. They are less likely to take part in recreational sports and more likely to cut back on their activity level once they have children.

Fortunately, research shows that you don't have to be an athlete to get mood benefits from exercise. Nor do you have to run, jog, lift weights, sweat, join a gym, buy special equipment, put on a skimpy leotard, or even change clothes. All you need to do is put on a pair of comfortable shoes, open the door, and start walking. Walk 10 minutes in one direction, turn around, and come back home. Midway into your first walk, you will begin to enjoy the "walker's high."

You probably know from personal experience that going for a walk can help you feel happier and less stressed, especially if you walk in a pleasant setting. But few people realize that a regular program of brisk walking is an even better way to enhance their mood than more intense exercise such as jogging or running. Until the 1990s, most of the scientists who were exploring

Raised to Look Cute

"I WAS RAISED TO LOOK cute in a tennis outfit and do country club sports. I was not raised to be physical."

LEVITY volunteer, 49

the link between mood and exercise focused on endorphins, so it was only natural that they study healthy young men performing strenuous feats. They had no idea that milder exercise can also enhance mood.

The first inkling came from surveys showing that people who were home gardeners or simply went for weekend walks were less likely to be depressed than more sedentary people. Slowly but surely, the researchers began shifting some of their focus from studying elite athletes running marathons to studying ordinary people doing ordinary things. *Out of this investigation has come the welcome finding that moderate-intensity exercise may be the best mood enhancer of all.*

Immediate Benefits of Your 20-Minute Brisk Walk

In recent years, researchers have learned a great deal about the way that moderate-intensity exercise stimulates the mind and body. Some of the changes take place within minutes. Imagine that you've just stepped out the door and started to walk. You are swinging your arms and aiming for a pace that is midway between a stroll and a jog. In just a minute or two, your heart begins to beat more rapidly. As your heart rate increases, more blood flows to your brain. The increased blood flow sends more fuel to your brain, which enhances your ability to think and concentrate. Ten to 15 minutes into your walk, your brain circulation has increased by as much as 50 percent.[2] On a positron emission tomography (PET) scan, your brain would be lighting up with brighter colors, indicating a greater level of activity. If you were given a test of intelligence and memory before and after your walk, you would score better after getting the exercise.[3]

At the same time that the brisk walk is stimulating your brain, it is also revving up your body. Walking releases some of the same activating substances that are triggered by stress. But the amounts generated by walking make you feel energized and alert, not tense and irritable.[4] In technical terms, researchers would say that walking produces an *energetic arousal* rather than a *tense arousal*. As you head for home, your mental fog is lifting, you feel more invigorated, and your mood has inched up several notches. The benefits continue even when you get home. For the next few hours, you will feel less anxious, happier, and more energetic.

Many women turn to food to experience these same good feelings. But walking is a much better way to generate a sustained sense of well-being. A current study compared the mood effects of eating a candy bar with going for a 10-minute brisk walk. When the volunteers ate the candy bars, they enjoyed a "sugar high" that lasted for about 30 minutes. But in less than an hour, they were feeling more tired and tense than they had before eating the sugary snack. When the same people went for a 10-minute walk, however, they felt good while they were taking their walk and continued to feel energized and more cheerful for several hours afterward with *no* dip in mood or energy level.[5] Candy gives you a short-term boost in mood, but brisk walking rewards you with hours of sustained contentment.

The Long-Term Benefits of Brisk Walking

A regular program of brisk walking also gives you even longer-lasting benefits. Once you've been walking for several weeks, you will have increased the activity of a number of mood-boosting substances. Most of our understanding of the way that exercise alters brain chemistry comes from animal studies. In a typical experiment, a colony of rats is divided into two equal groups. One group is given access to exercise wheels, and the other is not. After a few weeks, the researchers measure the brain chemicals in both groups of rats. Invariably, they find that the exercising rats have higher levels of serotonin, dopamine, and a third chemical messenger called norepinephrine—nature's antidepressants.[6]

It's important to note that the rats do not have to be exercising strenuously in order to have more of these chemicals. All they have to do is take a spin on the wheel whenever the spirit moves them. In fact, when the scientists *force* the rats to exercise by dropping the hapless creatures onto moving treadmills, the rats show classic signs of stress and lose some of their interest in sex.[7] In order to experience the full zest for life, they have to be exercising at a moderate pace of their own free will.

More recently, we've learned that the same phenomenon occurs in humans. In a study published in 2001, sedentary volunteers were asked to exercise moderately once a day for 3 weeks. At the end of the assignment, they had more serotonin receptors in their brains and a better mood. But when trained athletes were asked to exercise strenuously for 4 weeks, they had *fewer* serotonin receptors and a more depressed mood once the assignment was over.[8] The bottom line is that if you are exercising in order to improve your mood and relieve stress, moderate-intensity exercise is best.

The 20-Minute Solution

As my colleagues and I were planning the LEVITY study, we decided that brisk walking was the ideal exercise to include in our program. But we had a few unanswered questions: How long should we ask our volunteers to walk each day? How many days a week? Exactly how fast should they walk? One study in particular helped answer our questions. In this 1989 clinical trial, volunteers were assigned to one of three different types of exercise: (1) slow stretching for 30 minutes a day, (2) brisk walking for 20 minutes a day, or (3) jogging for 30 minutes a day.[9] The activities were designed to cover the spectrum from mild to moderately strenuous exercise.

After 10 weeks, the volunteers were given the usual physical and mental exams. As the researchers had expected, the joggers had become the most physically fit. But to their surprise, the joggers felt more tense and irritable than they had before the study began. The exercise had been so demanding on these formerly sedentary volunteers that it had created tense arousal rather than energetic arousal. The leisurely stretchers, meanwhile, showed virtually no change in mood. This is consistent with other studies that have shown that you need to be more active to get many mood benefits. Only one

Walking, Not Jogging, Lowers Tension and Confusion

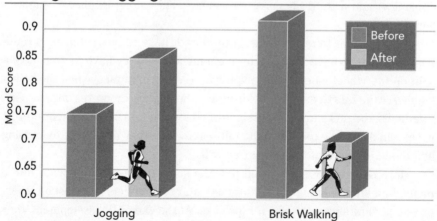

This graph of mood test scores shows how brisk walking and jogging influenced the mood of the volunteers. The higher the bar, the greater the tension. As you can see, the volunteers who jogged felt more tense and stressed at the end of the study, while those who went for brisk walks felt more calm and relaxed. (Data from Moses, Steptoe, et al. 1989. J. Psychosom. Res. 33 [1]: 47–61.)

group of exercisers felt noticeably better—the brisk walkers. After 10 weeks of regular walks, they felt less tense, anxious, and confused, and they were better able to cope with stress. Partly on the basis of this study, we decided to ask our volunteers to follow the same formula and go for 20-minute brisk walks, 5 days a week.

Stress Alone Can Trigger the Body Blues

One of the benefits of taking part in a regular program of brisk exercise is that you will find it easier to cope with stress. Being able to handle stress is a vital coping skill in today's world. A stressful lifestyle or even a single stressful event increases your risk of depression.

Sadly, many of the women in this country lead very stressful lives. Working mothers are among the most stressed. Currently, 73 percent of all women with school-age children work outside the home. When they come home after a hard day at work, many are still expected to shoulder most of the parenting, cooking, shopping, and cleaning responsibilities. If an aging parent becomes sick or injured, they are the most likely caregivers. As long as everything runs smoothly, many women can manage this high-wire balancing act. But if the pressure keeps building, they can lose their emotional balance and fall off the wire. For months or even years, they can go through their days feeling exhausted, mildly anxious, and stressed, while sleeping poorly and eating too much.

One of the volunteers I coached in the LEVITY study provides a classic example of the stress-induced Body Blues. When I first met 51-year-old Gwen, I could see that she had an easygoing disposition. She told me that she had had few problems with PMS in earlier years and had even sailed through perimenopause. She had the first intimations of the Body Blues about 3 years prior to joining our study.

At the time, she had a low-paying but rewarding job at a nonprofit organization. The job became more of a burden, however, when she was asked to take on added fund-raising duties, requiring her to go to several evening community meetings each week. Then her teenage son was invited to join a private basketball team, which meant that Gwen and her husband began driving him to extra practices, taking part in fund-raising efforts, and cheering him on during all the games and tournaments. These two changes left Gwen with very little free time, and she began comforting herself with frequent snacks, especially late at night as she struggled to catch up on all the day's chores.

But these stresses seemed trivial to Gwen when she learned that her mother had been diagnosed with terminal breast cancer. Gwen was very close to her mother and dreaded losing her. When her mother needed more care than her father could provide, Gwen invited both her parents to come live with her. "I didn't hesitate one minute," she told me. To find time to take care of everyone's needs, Gwen had to shorten her hours at work and accept a cut in pay, adding more financial strain on the household. Then, as her mother became progressively weaker, her father was diagnosed with congestive heart failure. As you can imagine, taking care of two ailing parents was like a full-time nursing job.

"I thought I was unflappable," Gwen said, "but I'm not." Despite the fact that she had been blessed with a secure childhood, a cheerful disposition, few hormonal difficulties, and a strong marriage, 3 years of mounting stress had succeeded in giving her the Body Blues.

When Gwen heard that we were looking for volunteers for the LEVITY study, she leapt at the chance. "I'm not doing so well on my own," she confessed. "I need help in turning things around." I'm glad to report that Gwen experienced great relief from taking part in the program. "I don't know if my stress level is way down or I'm just better able to cope," she told me in a follow-up interview. "But now my entire life feels more manageable. I feel like myself again."

How Exercise Stress-Proofs Your Brain

A diabolical animal study that took place in 1994 shows how effectively exercise can prevent stress from turning into depression. In this research project, a team of investigators subjected a colony of rats to a series of unpleasant, unpredictable events—a proven way to make animals depressed. One day, the rats would be deprived of food. The next, they would be given mild electric shocks. The day after that, they would have their tails pinched or their cages tilted, or they would be left in bright light 24 hours a day. After several weeks of this scientific form of torture, the rats showed all the typical signs of depression. They were more anxious and less active and inquisitive, and they spent more time alone.

Making the animals depressed was not the intent of this particular study, however. The goal was to see if exercise could *keep* stressed animals from becoming depressed. To find out, the investigators put another group of rodents through the very same ordeal. But this time, the rats were allowed to exercise each day before being subjected to the torture. At the end of 4 weeks,

Why Does Exercise Prevent Stress from Turning into Depression?

One of the negative effects of stress is that it depletes the body's store of serotonin. This is true for lab rats and humans alike. Studies show that when rats are allowed to exercise before being stressed, they develop supersensitive serotonin receptors.

These super receptors make better use of whatever serotonin is available. The end result is that rats that exercise before being stressed have just as much serotonin activity in their brains as rats that have not been stressed at all. You might liken the rats to a farmer who has been given half the usual amount of seed corn. If he takes great care in planting every seed, he can grow just as much corn as a farmer who has the full allotment of seeds but wastes half of it.

the scientists were surprised to see that every one of the rats was symptom-free.[10] *Exercise had broken the causal link between stress and depression.*

A human study that took place at Wake Forest University in Winston-Salem, North Carolina, shows that exercise can stress-proof women as well.[11] As in the rat study, the experimenters had to devise a reliable way to stress their 48 female volunteers. At first they considered asking the women to do "serial 7s," a mental arithmetic test that involves counting backward from 100 by 7s. (I can begin to sweat after subtracting the first 7. What *is* 93 minus 7?) But they decided this test was far too tame. They wanted the women's hearts to pound and their blood pressures to soar. They finally decided to subject them to many people's worst nightmare—extemporaneous public speaking.

When the women arrived at the lab, they had no idea what was in store for them. The research team measured their blood pressures and heart rates and gave them several mood tests. Then some of the women were asked to rest quietly for 40 minutes, while the others were escorted to a nearby room that was equipped with exercise bikes. The women were asked to pedal the bikes for about 30 minutes.

Then all the volunteers were assembled once again and given their dreaded assignment. They were told that each one of them would have to give an extemporaneous 3-minute speech on a controversial subject in front of two judges. The judges would be rating them on the organization and delivery of their talks. Someone else would be videotaping their talks, so their speeches could be scrutinized later for content and clarity. The best and worst speeches would be selected and used as examples. To make the women even more self-conscious, they were instructed to keep their hands still as they talked, enunciate clearly, and talk for the full 3 minutes. The women were then given their topics and allowed only 1 minute to prepare. A nightmare made real.

The intent of the study, of course, was not to see if the women were good extemporaneous speakers. The goal was to see if the women who had exercised before being given the assignment would be less stressed than the ones who had been resting quietly. The women were sent to individual rooms to give their talks. When the ordeal was finally over, they were given another round of physical and mood tests. As was true in the rat study, the women who had exercised before giving their talks responded much better to the pressure. They had a smaller increase in heart rate and blood pressure and fewer anxious thoughts.

Even a 20-minute exercise session can help buffer stress. In a 1989 study of college students, the volunteers were divided into an exercise group and a nonexercise group. After 20 minutes of either bicycling or resting, the students were given some complicated mental arithmetic. To heighten the stakes, they were told that their test results would be viewed as an accurate measure of their intelligence. As in the previous study, the students who had exercised before taking the test were less tense and anxious than those who had not.[12]

These findings about exercise and stress contain important lessons for all women. As was true for Gwen, you can't always lead a low-stress life. Some events are out of your control. For example, you might be laid off from work, discover you have a life-threatening illness, or lose someone you love. In addition to these unpredictable major stresses, there will be times when you *choose* to add more stress to your life. Like Gwen, for example, you might volunteer to care for your ailing parents even though it's going to make your life much more difficult. Or you might decide to go back to college to finish your degree even though you know you will feel more stressed for the next 2 years. You take on these added pressures because the activities are important enough to you to justify the stress.

She Copes Better with Stress

"NOW, WITH THE EXERCISE, my mood is more level. There's more equilibrium. When I do have these stresses in my work, personal life, whatever—I can deal with them without the big swings."

LEVITY volunteer, 31

But the good news is that you can take on these challenges and still maintain a level mood if you set aside the time to go for frequent brisk walks.

The Advantage of Being Outdoors

Walking will help relieve your stress and reduce your vegetative symptoms whether you do it on a treadmill indoors or go at a brisk pace outdoors. But an *outdoor* walk will be even more effective. Why? Being outside puts you in touch with the natural world. Whether you walk in a park in downtown Chicago or along the shore on Cape Cod, being outside brings you closer to the seasons and to nature.

This turned out to be important for many of our LEVITY volunteers. A woman who took her daily walks around her suburban neighborhood told us, "Nature isn't just a blur I see from my car window. I see how things change from day to day. This year, I got to see all the flowers as each one came into bloom." A 69-year-old woman who walked in the arboretum near her home said that her daily excursions made her aware of how few bird songs she recognized. She began packing along a bird book and binoculars. "Now I recognize more than a dozen bird calls," she told us, "and I've joined the local Audubon Society." A college art student began carrying a digital camera on her walks so that she could e-mail the photos to family members who lived in another state. "I wanted them to get a better sense of where I lived," she said. Even people who walked in downtown Seattle looked forward to their walks. They got to peer in shop windows, explore new streets, and feel the pulse of the city.

Exercising indoors is usually a more sterile experience. There you are on that same treadmill or exercise bike facing the same wall. Because you have fewer distractions, time seems to pass more slowly. You may be more aware of unpleasant sensations such as that soreness in your right calf or the labored sound of your own breathing. Having this internal focus can actually reduce the mood benefits you get from exercise.

In a 1995 study at James Cook University in Queensland, Australia, 10 trained athletes were sent on two 40-minute runs. One run was on a treadmill in the university gymnasium; the other was on a woodsy path that encircled the campus. The volunteers ran at the same pace for the same amount of time. When the athletes ran on the outdoor trail, their test scores showed that they felt more energetic and less anxious, depressed, angry, and hostile. When they ran on an indoor treadmill, however, their moods did not change for better or worse. What's more, they felt more fatigued after the run than they had before getting the exercise.[13] *From this and other studies, we know that the best way to improve mood is to exercise moderately for a comfortable period of time in an enjoyable location.*

I hasten to add that some people enjoy exercising indoors. Some love to exercise at the gym or take part in an indoor aerobics or dance class. I find that even working out on a stairclimber can be tolerable as long as I can read at the same time. But the bottom line is that you need to enjoy what you're doing. If exercising indoors makes you feel bored or restless or focuses your attention on unpleasant bodily sensations, you may not get all the mood benefits you are seeking.

Light Plus Exercise—An Unbeatable Combination

There's an even more important reason to walk outdoors whenever possible: You will be getting the combined benefits of daylight and exercise. I was surprised to learn what a difference combining exercise and

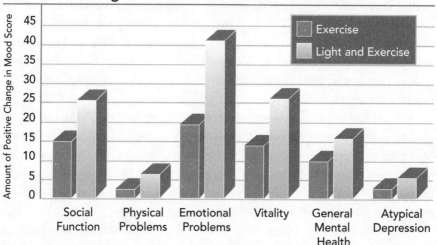

Exercise Plus Light Is Better Than Exercise Alone

In this graph, the height of the bars represents the degree of mood improvement in the two groups of volunteers. The dark bars represent the improvement in people who exercised under normal lighting conditions, and the taller, light-colored bars show the improvement in the people who exercised under bright light. As you can see, both groups benefited from their exercise programs, but the group that got both light and exercise felt markedly better. (Data from Partonen, Leppamaki, et al. 1998. Psychol. Med. 28 [6]: 1359–64. p. 1363.)

light can make. In the graph at the left, you can see the amount of mood improvement in people who exercised in a room with ordinary light (represented by the dark bars) versus those who exercised in bright light (represented by the light bars). The people who got both bright light and exercise felt markedly better than those who exercised under normal lighting conditions.[14] When you walk outdoors, you, too, will get to enjoy these heightened benefits.

Lose Fat and Feel Great

At the same time that going for frequent brisk walks will help relieve your stress and brighten your mood, it will also be burning excess calories. When you walk for just 20 minutes a day, 5 days a week, you will burn about 40,000 extra calories a year. At this rate, you can lose as much as 11 pounds per year—without dieting. Better yet, you will be losing fat, not muscle. The most effective way to burn fat is to exercise at 60 to 75 percent of your maximum heart rate, a level of intensity known as the fat-burning zone.[15] A brisk walk places you in this most favorable zone. Walking also tones your muscles, improves your posture, and gives you a more healthy, youthful appearance.

If you have a significant amount of weight to lose, however, you may not be content with such a slow, steady weight loss. One way to speed up the process is to lengthen your walks. Just make sure that going for longer walks does not make you feel pressured or stressed, which will be counterproductive for your mood. Another way to lose weight more quickly is to make a conscious effort to cut back on calories. Eating 500 fewer calories a day, which is a realistic goal for most women, can double your weight loss.

Fortunately, you are likely to find it much easier to restrain your eating once you have been on the LEVITY program for a few weeks. First, your mood will be improving day by day, so you will feel less compelled to turn to food for comfort and solace. Second, you will be feeling more energetic. Many of our volunteers told us that they felt so energized by the program that they began extending their walks or looking for additional ways to be active. Third, getting more daylight will help reduce your craving for carbohydrates—especially during the second half of the day.

But as soon as you start to experience these welcome changes in appetite and energy, it's important that you act on them. If you continue to eat the same amount of food out of habit or stick with your sedentary habits, it will take you much longer to lose weight. (For more information concerning how to lose weight on the LEVITY program, visit our Web site www.thebodyblues.com.)

The Long-Term Prognosis

Although walking gives you both short-term and long-term benefits, you will need to continue to exercise on a regular basis to keep enjoying all these rewards. This is why it's important to choose a type of exercise that you enjoy and will stick with. Many women like to go for walks, which is one of the reasons we chose this particular form of exercise for our program. We wanted our volunteers to continue to exercise and feel better long after the study was over.

This is exactly what happened. When we surveyed our LEVITY volunteers 1½ years after the completion of the study, 86 percent of the women who responded said that they were still going for outdoor walks, even though we had not been in contact with them during that entire time. A surprising 76 percent of them were walking three or more times a week. Even more gratifying to us was the fact that the women had also maintained their good moods. Eighty-nine percent of the women ranked their mood a 7 or higher on a scale of 1 to 10. The fact that they were still walking and still feeling great is a testimony to the effectiveness and appeal of the program.

The Positive "Side Effects" of Walking

Most pharmaceutical solutions to the Body Blues have a number of negative side effects. Walking has a few "side effects" as well, but they are uniformly positive. For example, regular brisk walking reduces your risk of cardiovascular disease, women's number one killer. Years ago, experts maintained that you had to exercise strenuously to benefit your heart. We now know from a study of 39,372 women that walking for just 1 hour a week *at any pace* cuts your risk of coronary heart disease in half.[16] (You will be exercising at least 1 hour and 40 minutes a week on the LEVITY program.) Other studies have shown that regular moderate-intensity exercise lowers your risk of stroke, diabetes, high blood pressure, osteoporosis, insomnia, obesity, and breast cancer.[17] Frequent walking may even add several years to your life.[18]

For these reasons, I recommend that my patients become regular walkers even if they don't have the Body Blues. The fact that walking also relieves vegetative symptoms of depression makes it my number one prescription.

Going for a brisk outdoor walk:

- Increases your serotonin and dopamine activity
- Increases your cerebral blood flow
- Reduces your tension and anxiety
- Raises your energy level
- Improves your ability to cope with stress
- Burns fat
- Decreases your appetite
- Connects you with nature
- Reduces your risk of a number of life-threatening diseases

Chapter 6

The Women's Antidepressant Cocktail

Six Inexpensive Vitamins and Minerals Proven to Boost Women's Mood

As you have seen, brightening your indoor environment and going for regular outdoor walks can jump-start the production of a number of mood-enhancing, stress-relieving, and appetite-suppressing chemicals. But your body cannot manufacture those chemicals unless it has the raw ingredients necessary to make them. The third and final component of the LEVITY program supplies these essential ingredients. When you add this antidepressant "cocktail" to a program of bright light and moderate-intensity exercise, you have a clinically proven solution for the Body Blues.

First, here's a quick overview of the six ingredients in the formula. Four of the ingredients are in the B-complex family. Many people think of the B vitamins as antistress vitamins, which is an apt description. Vitamin D, a fat-soluble vitamin, is the fifth ingredient. The final component is selenium, a trace mineral. All of these vitamins and minerals are inexpensive and can be found at most grocery stores and pharmacies. The cost of the entire cocktail is about 25 cents a day. (For the purposes of our study, we asked a company to produce a supplement that contains all of the ingredients in one easy-to-swallow tablet. The LEVITY™ Mood-Elevating Formula can be found at your local health food store, pharmacy, or supermarket, or turn to page 160 for ordering information. Neither my coauthor nor I benefit from the sale of the supplements.)

Why a Formula Just for Women?

Although the LEVITY formula can boost the mood of men as well as women, it is likely to be more beneficial for women. The main reason is that we designed it specifically to meet women's needs. For example, one factor that influenced our choice of ingredients is that women are more likely than men to be deficient in certain nutrients, especially the B vitamins. Their lower intake of the B vitamins is partly due to the fact that more women than men are on diets low in these key nutrients, including low-calorie, vegetarian, and vegan diets. Taking oral contraceptives and perhaps hormone replacement therapy can also increase the need for vitamin B_6.

Another and more surprising reason that the LEVITY formula is likely to work better for women is that some of the ingredients have been shown to improve the mood or mental performance of women but not men. One of the people who helped uncover these gender differences is David Benton, Ph.D., professor and researcher at the University College of Wales. In 1995, Dr. Benton and his colleagues gave multivitamin supplements or look-alike placebos to 127 healthy young men and women for a period of 1 year. (Four of the ingredients in his supplement—vitamins B_1, B_2, B_6, and folic acid—are included in the LEVITY formula.) At the end of the study, the women taking the vitamins performed better on a range of mental tests, while the men showed no such improvement.[1] Studies like Dr. Benton's suggest that men and women not only have different mood issues, they also respond differently to the same therapies. Gender matters.

> # The LEVITY Formula
>
> To experience the full benefits of the LEVITY program, take the following amounts of these six vitamins and minerals every day.
>
> - 50 milligrams vitamin B_1 (thiamin)
> - 50 milligrams vitamin B_2 (riboflavin)
> - 50 milligrams vitamin B_6 (pyridoxine)
> - 400 micrograms* folic acid
> - 400 IU vitamin D_3 (cholecalciferol)
> - 200 micrograms selenium
>
> *A microgram is one millionth of a gram.

Vitamins as Mood Therapy

The fact that high doses of certain vitamins and minerals can improve mood and cognition is a relatively new discovery. Until the mid-20th century, vitamins and minerals were viewed as substances needed to prevent serious diseases, such as scurvy, pellagra, beriberi, and rickets. Because it took only small amounts of the nutrients to prevent or treat these diseases, it was assumed that you could get all you needed from eating a well-balanced diet.

About 30 or so years ago, scientists began investigating whether taking higher doses of certain nutrients might offer some added health benefits. At first, the research was limited to preventing diseases such as cancer, heart disease, and diabetes. But in the 1990s, a few researchers, including Dr. Benton, began exploring the effects of high-dose supplements on mood. It is ironic that it took so long for scientists to investigate the vitamin/mood connection, because the first signs of vitamin deficiency are often mental, emotional, or cognitive changes. For instance, a deficiency in certain B vitamins can make you feel depressed, apprehensive, and irritable long before you are aware of any physical changes.

The nutrient/mood research is still in its infancy. But enough reliable information exists about the safety and effectiveness of the six ingredients in the LEVITY formula that we decided to make them an integral part of our program. In this chapter, I will talk about some of those key findings.

The Six LEVITY Ingredients

Vitamin B_1 (Thiamin)

Fifty milligrams of vitamin B_1, commonly known as thiamin, is the first of the six ingredients in the LEVITY formula. A few years after Dr. Benton con-

---

How Vitamin B_1 Relieves Fatigue and Improves Your Memory

One of the ways that vitamin B_1, also known as thiamin, influences your mood is by protecting your nerve fibers and the structure that surrounds them called the myelin sheath. An extreme lack of this vitamin can result in Korsakoff's psychosis, a mental condition in which people become apathetic and have difficulty forming new memories. Taking B_1 supplements brings about a dramatic recovery.

Vitamin B_1 is also involved in the production of acetylcholine, a chemical that helps your brain store and retrieve information. (Some people refer to acetylcholine as the "ink" in your mental note-taking system. When you run out of ink, you can't record any more memories.) Women who have even a mild deficiency of B_1 are more likely to have memory problems than women with adequate levels. Fatigue is another common symptom of B_1 deficiency. Without vitamin B_1, you cannot metabolize proteins or carbohydrates, depriving you of these essential sources of energy. Finally, animal studies show that vitamin B_1 helps activate serotonin, perhaps by making it easier to bind to its receptors.

Vitamin B₁ Improves Mood in Women

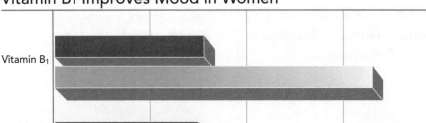

This graph shows the difference in mood between women who took vitamin B_1 and those who took a placebo. The dark bars show the average mood of the women before the study began. The light bars show their mood 2 months later. The longer the bars, the better the women's mood. As you can see, the women who took vitamin B_1 felt significantly better than those who took the placebos. (Data from Benton, Griffiths, and Haller 1997. Psychopharmacology 129: 66–71.)

ducted his multivitamin study mentioned above, he decided to see if any of the ingredients in his formula had been more effective than others. The preliminary evidence pointed to vitamin B_1. To test the theory, he gave tablets containing 50 milligrams of B_1 or look-alike placebos to a group of healthy young women. Despite the fact that none of the women had been deficient in the vitamin before the study began, those taking the supplement felt more clearheaded, energetic, and composed in just 2 months.[2] Other studies have shown that vitamin B_1 can help older women sleep better at night and feel more energetic during the day[3] and can also enhance the effectiveness of antidepressants.[4]

Certain women are more likely to be low in B_1 than others, including vegetarians, vegans, older women in general (as many as 90 percent may be deficient in B_1), alcoholics, cocaine users, women on high-carbohydrate diets, and women with HIV/AIDS, anorexia nervosa, chronic fatigue syndrome, or Alzheimer's disease.

You can get an adequate amount of B_1 (as defined by the USDA) by eating a diet that includes meat (especially pork), yeast, legumes, whole grains, or

Vitamin B₂ Is Required to Produce Mood-Boosting Chemicals

Vitamin B₂, also known as riboflavin, helps your body metabolize proteins, fats, and carbohydrates. It is also involved in red blood cell formation (which plays a role in energy production) and helps with the absorption of iron and the metabolism of vitamin B₆. In addition, vitamin B₂ is essential for the production of serotonin, norepinephrine, and dopamine.

enriched cereals and breads. It would be very difficult, however, to get the full 50 milligrams without taking a dietary supplement.

Vitamin B₂ (Riboflavin)

Fifty milligrams of vitamin B₂, also known as riboflavin, is the second ingredient in the LEVITY formula. In Dr. Benton's multivitamin study mentioned earlier, women who had an improved vitamin B₂ status had a more agreeable mood, better composure, and clearer thinking. A study by another investigator found that giving vitamin B₂ to older people who are taking antidepressants makes the drugs more effective.[5]

Older women have a high risk of being deficient in B₂. A current British study found that a staggering 78 percent of women ages 68 to 90 had too little of the vitamin.[6] Pregnant women, women on high-protein diets, vegetarians, and vegans are also more likely to be low in B₂.

Good dietary sources of vitamin B₂ include meat (especially organ meats), poultry, yeast, wheat germ, dairy products, soybeans, bran, fatty fish, dark green leafy vegetables, almonds, and B₂-enriched products. As is true for B₁, however, it is difficult to get 50 milligrams of vitamin B₂ from food sources alone.

Vitamin B₆ (Pyridoxine)

This vitamin has been called the "women's vitamin" because it helps treat a number of conditions unique to women, including PMS, nausea during pregnancy, and the side effects of taking oral contraceptives or hormone replacement therapy.

One reason B₆ is so beneficial for women is that it is essential for the production of serotonin, the brain's primary feel-good chemical. In one small German study, men and women given 80 milligrams of vitamin B₆ each night for a period of a week had higher levels of serotonin than those who were given placebos.[7]

Vitamin B₆ also helps create a type of fat that may have mood-enhancing effects. The human brain is 60 percent fat, and one of the most important fats

Taking Vitamin B₆ Increases Serotonin

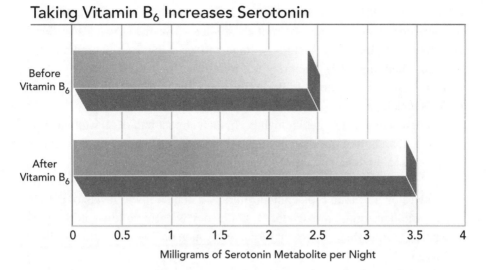

The two bars above show the serotonin levels in volunteers before and after taking relatively high doses of vitamin B₆. Taking this one vitamin alone caused a significant increase in the mood-elevating brain chemical. (Data from Demisch and Kaczmarczyk 1991. Adv. Exp. Med. Biol. 294: 519–22.)

in the brain is called DHA (docosahexaenoic acid, a type of omega-3 fatty acid). People with low levels of DHA are more likely to be depressed.[8] Researchers at the National Institute of Mental Health are investigating whether DHA can treat a number of disorders, including depression, bipolar disorder (formerly known as manic-depressive disorder), and attention deficit hyperactivity disorder.

The most common way to increase your intake of DHA is by eating fatty fish (tuna, trout, salmon, mackerel, sardines) or by taking fish-oil capsules. But you can also increase the amount of DHA in your brain simply by taking more vitamin B₆. When you have enough of this B vitamin, your body is able to make DHA from another omega-3 fatty acid, called alpha-linolenic acid, found in walnuts, flaxseeds, dark green leafy vegetables, products from animals raised in pastures, and canola oil.

Given the many ways that B₆ influences your brain chemistry, it is not surprising that taking this one vitamin alone may relieve some of the symptoms of the Body Blues. Dr. Benton found that giving vitamin B₆ to women helped them think more clearly.[9] South African researchers discovered that B₆ improved the mood of depressed college students.[10] Children who were given B₆ at night produced more melatonin, the body's sleep-inducing hormone.[11] It is possible that B_6 boosts melatonin in adults as well, helping to promote deeper sleep. Some, but not all, studies show that B_6 can also relieve symptoms of PMS. In a 1989 study, women with premenstrual symptoms who took 50 milligrams of B_6 each day felt less tired, depressed, and irritable.[12] Women who have the monthly Body Blues are likely to find the LEVITY formula especially helpful.

Many women do not get enough B_6. In fact, almost half of all women consume less than half of the Daily Value (DV) of vitamin B_6. Some of the women most likely to be deficient are older women in general, athletes, vegetarians, heavy drinkers, and women with chronic fatigue syndrome. Taking oral contraceptives or hormone replacement therapy can also lower levels of the vitamin. Another common cause of B_6 deficiency is eating a low-calorie diet. One survey found that 75 percent of young women on calorie-restricted diets are deficient in B_6.[13]

Good food sources of B_6 include meat (especially chicken and pork), beans (especially chickpeas), cereals, brown rice, potatoes, bananas, sunflower seeds, peanut butter, and vitamin-fortified products. But you are not likely to consume the recommended 50 milligrams without taking a supplement.

You need to be cautious when taking high doses of vitamin B_6, however. Some people who have taken 500 milligrams or more for longer than 2 years have developed neuropathy, sensory nerve damage. (Five hundred milligrams is 10 times the amount in the LEVITY formula.) To be safe, the USDA has set the tolerable upper limit, or UL, for B_6 at 100 milligrams. (The UL can be thought of as the highest daily intake over a prolonged time known to pose no risks to most members of a healthy population.) In order to stay below this level, do not combine the LEVITY formula with other supplements high in B_6.

People with diabetes should consult their health care providers before taking 50 milligrams of B_6, because the vitamin can lower blood sugar. Those taking levodopa (L-dopa) or anticonvulsant medications should also consult their

---

Vitamin B_6 Helps Convert Tryptophan into Serotonin

Your body makes serotonin from an amino acid (a protein fragment) called tryptophan, which is abundant in your food. But in order to reshape tryptophan into serotonin, you need an enzyme called decarboxylase, which is dependent upon vitamin B_6. Taking extra vitamin B_6 increases your supply of this enzyme, thereby stimulating serotonin production.

health care providers before taking supplemental B$_6$, because the vitamin can reduce the effectiveness of those drugs.

Folic Acid

The fact that folic acid enhances people's moods has received very little attention, despite a wealth of positive data. First of all, it has been known for decades that depressed people have low levels of folic acid. One survey determined that as many as 38 percent of all depressed people are deficient in this vitamin. The lower the level, the more severe their depression.[14] The link between depression and low folic acid levels has been called "one of the most robust findings in the biochemistry of major depression."[15]

A recent finding is that folic acid may have a major impact on how well depressed women respond to antidepressants. In a study published in 2000, depressed men and women who were taking Prozac were given either 500 micrograms of folic acid or a placebo. Ninety-three percent of the women given the folic acid responded well to the combined treatment, compared with only 61 percent of the women given Prozac and a placebo. The researchers concluded: "Folic acid is a simple method of greatly improving the antidepressant action of fluoxetine [Prozac] and probably other antidepressants."[16] Significantly, the men who took folic acid and Prozac showed no improvement over those given placebos.

In a small but compelling study, depressed older patients were given folic acid without any other medication. Eighty-one percent of the patients experienced substantial relief, which is a greater percentage than typically responds to antidepressant drugs.[17]

Folic acid deficiency was very common until 1998 when the U.S. government mandated that folic acid be added to enriched flour and cereals. Prior to that time, the average intake was only 242 micrograms, which is a little more than half of the DV of 400 micrograms. Fortifying cereals and flour has added an estimated 100 micrograms, but this means that most Americans are still below the recommended amount.

Women most likely to be deficient in folic acid include those who are age 60 and older and those who have chronic fatigue syndrome, rheumatoid arthritis, alcohol dependency, cancer, or HIV/AIDS. Black and Latina women are also at greater risk.

Food sources highest in folate (the natural form of folic acid) are brewer's yeast, liver, kidney, orange juice, green leafy vegetables, fortified grain products, dried beans and peas, and most berries. The UL for folic acid is 1,000 micrograms. (This is more than twice the amount in the

Folic Acid Helps Relieve Depression

One of the ways that folic acid enhances your mood is by helping your body produce more of a natural antidepressant known as s-adenosylmethionine, or SAM-e (pronounced "Sammy"). In recent years, SAM-e has been available in supplement form and has become a popular over-the-counter remedy for depression. There is good reason for its widespread use. Several small studies have shown that SAM-e works as well as conventional antidepressant medications—only more quickly and with fewer side effects. To make sure that your body is making enough of its own SAM-e, you need an adequate intake of folic acid. Two other components required for the production of SAM-e are vitamin B_6 and selenium. All three are included in the LEVITY formula.

M. I. Botez, Ph.D., of the Clinical Research Institute of Montreal, found that depressed patients with signs of folic acid deficiency also had low serotonin levels. What's more, some of the patients who were treated with folic acid produced almost twice as much serotonin and experienced significant relief from their symptoms. Interestingly, 90 percent of the people who were responsive to the treatment were women.[18]

LEVITY formula.) People who are taking anticonvulsant medications should consult their primary care providers before taking folic acid supplements. Currently, many pregnant women are taking 600 micrograms of folic acid. Taking additional amounts is not advised without your practitioner's approval.

One of the "side effects" of folic acid is that it can help prevent birth defects. It also lowers the levels of homocysteine, a chemical in the blood that increases your risk of cardiovascular disease. (High levels of homocysteine can damage the cells that line your heart and arteries.) In fact, women who have high blood levels of both folic acid and vitamin B_6 have a 45 percent lower risk of developing coronary heart disease.[19] The LEVITY formula contains both of these nutrients. So in addition to boosting your mood and energy level, the supplement may put you in the lowest risk category for heart disease.

Vitamin D_3 (Cholecalciferol)

Our natural source of vitamin D is the sun. When ultraviolet (UV) light from the sun falls on our bare skin, it interacts with a type of fat (7-dehydrocholesterol) that is eventually converted into vitamin D. Because our sun exposure tends to follow a seasonal pattern, vitamin D levels peak in the summer and then begin to decline in autumn. The lowest levels of vitamin D typically occur in late winter. The graph below shows the average levels of vitamin D in healthy adults living in Michigan.[20] As you can see, their vitamin D levels were highest from May through September.

Is it a coincidence that most people's moods tend to peak in the summer and sink in the winter? Not according to Allen Lansdowne, Ph.D., a researcher from the department of psychology at the University of Newcastle in Australia. Dr. Lansdowne theorized that one reason people have winter depression is that they've run out of their summer store of vitamin D, which has proven mood-elevating properties.

To test his theory, Dr. Lansdowne and his colleagues gave vitamin D supplements or placebos to 34 women and 10 men during Australia's winter months. In only 5 days, the volunteers given the vitamin D had a much better mood than those given placebos. In fact, most of them reported that they were feeling "really good" for the entire 5 days, a sentiment shared by none of those who were taking placebos. (See "Vitamin D Boosts Mood in Winter" on page 94.)[21]

Eons ago, when our ancestors spent the majority of their time outdoors,

Vitamin D Levels Peak in Summer

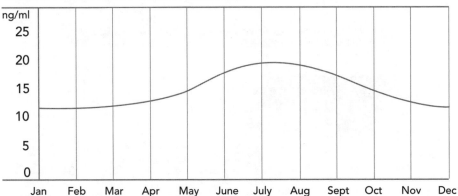

The gentle curve on this graph shows how vitamin D levels (measured in nanograms per milliliter) increase from April to October, the months when people get the most sunlight and also tend to have the best moods. In the winter, people have relatively low levels of the vitamin, which could be one of the underlying causes of seasonal affective disorder and the less severe winter blues. (Data from Stryd, Gilbertson, et al. 1979. J. Clin. Endocrinol. Metab. 48 [5]: 771–5.)

a deficiency of vitamin D would have been physically impossible. Exposing your entire body to sunlight for about an hour is equivalent to taking 10,000 IU of vitamin D—25 times the recommended dose. The only reason early humans did not accumulate toxic amounts of the vitamin is that sunlight both creates and breaks down vitamin D, maintaining a healthy balance.

Today, however, we've moved indoors. When we do venture outside, we are advised to cover our bodies with clothing or slather ourselves with sunscreen. (A sunscreen with an SPF greater than 8 blocks vitamin D production.)[22] Many people do not get enough sun on their bare skin to create even the minimum amount of vitamin D required for good health.

To gain more insight into what happens to vitamin D levels when people avoid the sun, the U.S. Navy measured the vitamin levels of a submarine crew before and after they went on a 2-month undersea cruise. Although the crewmen were consuming the usual vitamin D–fortified milk and cereal products, their vitamin D levels were cut almost in half.[23]

Surprisingly, some older women have even lower levels of vitamin D than these sun-deprived sailors. As women age, their skin produces about one-

Vitamin D Boosts Mood in Winter

This graph illustrates the much better mood of the people who took vitamin D compared with those who took placebos. As in all studies of this nature, no one, not even the investigators, knew who was getting the real vitamin and who was getting the look-alike placebo. The longer the bar, the better the people's mood. (Data from Lansdowne and Provost 1998. Psychopharmacology [Berl] 135 [4]: 319–23.)

Vitamin D Stimulates the Production of Serotonin

You have vitamin D receptors everywhere in your body, including in a critical area of your brain (the dorsal raphe nucleus) that is part of the serotonin system. Vitamin D, like the B vitamins, stimulates the production or release of serotonin, perhaps by regulating calcium flow to the cells. The fact that taking the Daily Value (DV) of vitamin D can improve mood in just 5 days, as was shown in Dr. Allen Lansdowne's study, suggests that the effect is a strong one indeed.

---

quarter as much vitamin D as it did when they were younger. Women of color are also likely to be low in vitamin D. The more pigmented your skin, the more slowly you create vitamin D. Light-skinned people can create an adequate amount of vitamin D with only 20 minutes of direct sun exposure. Dark-skinned people take almost 2 hours longer to produce the same amount. As a result, African-American women have only one-half the amount of vitamin D in their blood as Caucasians.[24]

Women living in the northern half of the United States also have an increased risk of vitamin D deficiency. In the winter months, the sun sinks lower toward the horizon in the north than it does in the south, so the rays of the sun have to penetrate more layers of the atmosphere. The atmosphere filters out much of the UV light, resulting in a lower production of vitamin D. People living in New York, Boston, Seattle, or Chicago, for example, produce little or no vitamin D from November through February, even on the sunniest days. All of their vitamin D must come from fortified products or from their dwindling summer supply.[25] The "vitamin D winter" can extend from October to March in Canada and parts of northern Europe.

Other women who are more likely to be deficient in this mood-enhancing vitamin are vegans (due to their avoidance of vitamin D–fortified milk products), women who work the night shift (and therefore see little daylight), people who cover their skin with sunscreen or are fully clothed whenever they go outdoors, and women who clothe their entire bodies for religious reasons. All told, at least one out of every seven adults is deficient in vitamin D.

There are only three reliable dietary sources of vitamin D: cod liver oil, fatty fish, and vitamin D–fortified milk. Since the 1930s, vitamin D has been added to milk in order to prevent rickets. (There is approximately 400 IU of vitamin D per quart.) But cheese, yogurt, and ice cream are rarely fortified.

Many women and girls drink less milk than they did in the past, because they have switched to soy milk, have food allergies, or want to cut calories.

An adequate intake (AI) of vitamin D for women is 200 IU for ages 19 to 50, 400 IU for ages 51 to 69, and 600 IU for those 70 and older. The Food and Nutrition Board of the Institute of Medicine has set the UL for vitamin D at 2,000 IU. (*Note:* This is five times the amount in the LEVITY formula.)

Selenium

Dr. David Benton, the pioneering British researcher mentioned earlier, has proven that the trace mineral selenium also has mood-elevating properties. In 1990, he gave 100 micrograms of selenium or a placebo to 17 men and 33 women. Those taking the selenium felt less anxious, less depressed, and more energetic in just 2½ weeks. Their moods continued to improve during the next few weeks.[26]

Why did selenium have such a dramatic effect on the volunteers' moods? A new finding is that selenium may enhance the dopamine activity in the brain, increasing the sense of arousal and pleasure.[27] As you learned in chapter 2, women have low dopamine activity whenever they have low or falling estrogen levels. Taking selenium can help compensate for this reduction and relieve some of the symptoms of the Body Blues.

Selenium Improves Mood in 2½ Weeks

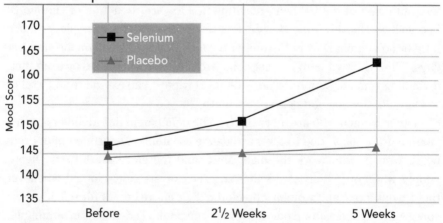

This graph shows the marked improvement in mood in the people who took 100 micrograms of selenium (the black line) and the lack of change in those taking the placebo. Those taking the selenium felt less depressed and more energetic in 2½ weeks. (Data from Benton and Cook 1990. Psychopharmacology 102 [4]: 549–50.)

In addition to improving your mood, selenium may also reduce the risk of cancer. In a study published in the *Journal of the American Medical Association* in 1996, men and women with a history of skin cancer were given either a placebo or 200 micrograms of selenium. (This is the same amount as in the LEVITY formula.) The goal of the study was to see if the trace mineral could prevent further skin cancers. After 10 years, there was no difference in the number of new skin cancers between the groups. To everyone's surprise, however, there was a striking reduction in other types of cancer, including lung and colorectal cancer—two of the three most life-threatening cancers in women.[28]

The UL for selenium has been set at 400 micrograms per day—twice the amount in the LEVITY formula. The lowest level that has been found to cause adverse effects is 910 micrograms. Nonetheless, you should not take other supplements high in selenium while taking the LEVITY formula.

The Benefits of the LEVITY Supplement

As you have seen, the six ingredients in the LEVITY formula play an important role in relieving the Body Blues. When taken in the amounts recommended in the formula, they have been shown to have all the benefits listed below. Costing just 25 cents a day, the LEVITY supplement is a bargain indeed.

- Increased serotonin and dopamine production
- Increased feelings of clearheadedness and composure
- Higher energy level
- Fewer symptoms of PMS (in some women)
- Enhanced effectiveness of prescription antidepressants
- Relief from the symptoms of winter depression
- Reduced risk of cancer and cardiovascular disease

PART 3

How to Follow the LEVITY Program

Chapter 7

Bring Back the Light
Creating a More Natural Lighting Environment

This chapter gives you practical advice for creating a more natural lighting environment—the first of the three LEVITY activities. As I explained earlier, there are three ways that bright light can help relieve the Body Blues. First, when sunlight falls on your bare skin, you create more vitamin D, which has proven mood-elevating properties. But since you will be taking vitamin D as a daily supplement, you will not need to make a special effort to expose your skin to the sun. You can use sunscreen or cover your entire body with clothing and still get all the benefits of this important vitamin.

The second way that light influences your mood is by entering your eyes and triggering increased production of a variety of feel-good chemicals. Third, when bright light enters your eyes, you have greater blood flow to your brain, which helps you concentrate and remember. (I will be talking about ways to protect your eyes from ultraviolet light later on in this chapter.) The LEVITY program relies on these last two mechanisms.

Fine-Tuning the Amount of Light That Enters Your Eyes

As you know, one of the main ways you will be getting more light during the day is by taking an outdoor walk. There is more light available to you outdoors on a sunny day than in any other circumstance, including sitting in front of a 10,000-lux light box. On gray days, there is still enough light outdoors to brighten your mood.

The only disadvantage of using outdoor light to boost your mood is that light levels outdoors can vary from 1,000 lux on a very dark and cloudy day

LEVITY Gave Encouragement

"THE LEVITY STUDY ENCOURAGED me and motivated me to get out and walk during the daylight hours. I realized how much light means to me! The other day I put my face directly in the sun. It wasn't for color; it was just to feel great. The sun is so helpful."

LEVITY volunteer, 63

to 75,000 lux or more on a sunny day. One thousand lux is enough light to improve your mood, but more would be better. (Keep in mind that most indoor spaces have 200 lux or less.) Seventy-five thousand lux, however, is *more* light than you need to relieve your symptoms and can also seem too bright or glaring.

There are simple and effective ways to regulate the amount of light that enters your eyes. If it's cloudy outside or you are walking early or late in the day, look for ways to increase your light exposure. One way to do this is to plan your walk so that you are away from the shadows of tall buildings or trees and facing the sun rather than walking away from it.

Wherever you walk, look straight ahead rather than down at the ground (except as needed for safety). If you keep a level gaze, you can more than double the amount of light that enters your eyes. If you glance at the brightest part of the sky from time to time, you will get even more mood-boosting light. Silver linings *do* exist, and they do help brighten your mood. Think of the sky as your no-cost, energy-efficient light box. (Of course, *never* look directly at the sun. You can absorb enough ultraviolet light to damage your eyes in less than a minute.)

The surface that you walk on also influences your light exposure. Concrete bounces back more light than darker colored surfaces such as grass, dirt, or asphalt. Walking close to a body of water is an even better amplifier, giving you twice the light you would get walking in another location. For maximum benefits, look at the water as often as possible. (Here in Seattle, thousands of people walk around Green Lake every day, not knowing that they are getting a double helping of mood-boosting light.)

Walking in the rain presents a special challenge because the clouds block much of the light. But you diminish the light even more if you wear a broad-brimmed hat or an overhanging hood or use an ordinary opaque umbrella. To keep dry but still benefit from the light, wear a hood or hat that does not project over your eyes. Another rainy-day solution is to use a transparent umbrella. A see-through umbrella protects both you and your clothes but doesn't block the light. (We had to search far and wide to find a source of large, high-quality transparent umbrellas for our LEVITY volunteers. For ordering information, see page 169 of our resource section or visit www.thebodyblues.com.)

On bright, sunny days or when the ground is covered with snow, you will want to *reduce* your light exposure. (Snow can quadruple the amount of light that enters your eyes.) For eye comfort, wear sunglasses, walk in shadier areas, turn your back to the sun, look down at the ground, wear a brimmed hat, or walk early in the day or late in the afternoon. You will still be getting enough bright light to improve your energy level and mood.

> ## Even a Cloudy Day Helps
>
> "LAST SUMMER I WAS basically indoors. And you just become kind of a hermit, closed in. It's very easy to get depressed doing that. But getting out, even on a cloudy day, it really helps."
>
> **LEVITY volunteer, 71**

Let in the Good, but Block the Bad

Although you want to seek out the light, you do *not* want to compromise your eyesight by absorbing too much ultraviolet (UV) light. A natural, invisible component of sunlight, UV light increases your risk of a number of serious eye conditions, including cataracts and macular degeneration, the leading cause of blindness in adults. The more UV light that enters your eyes, the greater your risk.

The obvious solution is to wear sunglasses. Wraparound sunglasses offer the greatest protection. Look for sunglasses that receive an ANSI rating of at least 99 percent UVB protection and 98 percent UVA protection. Although polarized lenses reduce glare, the polarization itself does not block UV light.

Unfortunately, sunglasses do more than block harmful UV light. They also filter out 80 to 90 percent of the *visible* light as well—the very light you need to create mood-enhancing chemicals. To protect your eyes and still beat the Body Blues, wear lightly tinted or even clear sunglasses except in the brightest conditions. Contrary to popular belief, the tint in sunglasses blocks very little of the UV light. The solar protection comes from the lens material itself or from a clear film that is applied to the surface of the lens. The tint is added to reduce glare.

When you are shopping for sunglasses, hold them up to the light and choose the pair that lets in the most light. A few manufacturers offer clear, UV-shielded sunglasses (primarily for cyclists), but you won't find them at your local shopping mall. I did, however, recently discover a surprising source of inexpensive clear, UV-protected lenses—my local hardware store.

Ultraviolet Radiation

Ultraviolet (UV) radiation is short-wavelength radiation from 100 to 400 nanometers (nm) that makes up about 2 percent of the total solar energy that reaches the earth. UV light is further divided into three subcategories: UVA (315 to 380 nm), UVB (290 to 315 nm), and UVC (200 to 290 nm).

Most of the UVC is blocked by the atmosphere, so it is of little concern. Both UVA and UVB, however, penetrate the protective ozone layer. UVB is believed to be the most damaging to your eyes, although UVA light penetrates more deeply and can damage the retina. Therefore, you need to guard against both types, especially now that the thinning ozone layer allows greater transmission of UV light from 288 to 340 nm, which is all of the UVB range and much of the UVA.

Hardware stores carry special safety glasses designed to protect the eyes from flying debris. Some of the glasses are made from polycarbonate, a plastic that blocks 100 percent of the UV light. Although safety glasses are not designed to be worn as sunglasses and do not have that "Armani" look, they block UV light very well. Some cost less than $15. For the best optics, however, look for more expensive models.

For the highest-quality optics and a more fashionable look, order custom sunglasses from your optometrist. Explain that you want a very light tint. Optometrists refer to the lightest tint as a "number one tint." Clear lenses are referred to as "water clear." (The downside of lightly tinted glasses is that they do not block much of the glare, so you may squint on very bright days. Squinting, as you know, can give you crow's-feet.)

If you have sensitive eyes and need to reduce the glare or if you live in a sunny climate and get a great deal of sunlight, by all means wear sunglasses with a darker tint. But make an effort to match the tint to the available light. One way to do this is to buy *photochromic*, or changeable, sunglasses that darken when you are in bright light but become almost clear on a cloudy day. (Most changeable sunglasses block about 85 percent of the visible light on sunny days but only 10 to 15 percent on cloudy days.) Another alternative is to purchase two pairs of sunglasses—one for gray days and one for brighter conditions. Reserve very dark sunglasses, known as glacier glasses, for those times when you are walking in the snow, climbing at high altitude, boating, or skiing.

What about lens color? Alas, rose-colored glasses do not seem to improve your mood. A yellow tint might, however, simply because it lets in more light. Yellow lenses also improve visual contrast, which can be helpful for aging eyes. For the most accurate color perception, choose lenses with a light gray, blue, or brown tint.

Increase the UV Protection from Your Glasses and Contact Lenses

Few people realize that prescription glasses made from glass filter out all of the UVB light and some of the UVA light, simply because ordinary glass happens to absorb light in these particular spectrums. (Some surveys show that lifelong wearers of glasses have a lower risk of cataracts.) To increase the protection factor of your prescription glasses, ask your optometrist to apply an invisible coating that blocks UV light. (I've had this done to my own glasses. It's very affordable.) Plastic lenses offer varying degrees of UV protection. Those made from polycarbonate block 100 percent of the UV light, making them an ideal choice. (They are also lightweight and shatter resistant.) Ask your optometrist about UV protection when you are ordering your next pair of glasses.

Many types of contact lenses—including some of the newer disposable kinds—also block UV light to one degree or another. Contacts protect your eyes from sunlight coming from above and to the side better than all but the most face-hugging sunglasses. (Of course, no contact lens protects the entirety of your eye, nor your eyelids.) Rigid gas-permeable lenses block more UV light than soft lenses, but they cover less of your cornea. (You may have UV-blocking contact lenses already. Ask your optometrist.) Your optometrist will know which brands offer the most protection.

Shield Yourself—From the Inside Out

Finally, no matter what type of glasses you wear, it would be wise to apply some "internal sunblock" as well. The primary way that UV light damages your eyes and skin is by generating reactive molecules called free radicals that can damage healthy cells. Eating a diet that is rich in antioxidants and certain other nutrients helps prevent this damage. As an added bonus, when you increase your internal sunblock, you protect your entire body, not just your eyes, from free radical damage.

A Recipe for Your Internal Sunscreen

Add more of the following foods or supplements to your daily diet, and you will be boosting your invisible protection against ultraviolet light.

Bilberry
Carrots
Citrus fruits
Dark green leafy vegetables
Egg yolks
Folic acid supplements (included in the LEVITY formula)

Grapes
Green tea or green tea extract
Kale
Kiwifruit
Orange peppers
Selenium supplements (included in the LEVITY formula)
Spinach
Vitamin B_2 supplements (included in the LEVITY formula)
Vitamin C supplements
Vitamin E supplements

Three of the vitamins in the LEVITY formula have been proven to protect your eyes—selenium,[1] vitamin B_2 (riboflavin), and folic acid.[2] This means they will be doing double duty—helping to fight the Body Blues and shielding you from UV light. Other eye-protecting nutrients include vitamins C and E,[3] plus many of the carotenoids, such as beta-carotene, lutein, zeaxanthin, and lycopene. Green tea is also a proven UV protector.

Making the Most of Exercising Indoors

I recommend that you walk outdoors whenever possible, but there will be times when it is not practical. In the wintertime, for example, it may be dark when you go to work and dark when you come home, making it very difficult to walk outside during daylight hours. Or there may be times when it's too hot, wet, windy, slippery, or cold for it to be wise to go outdoors.

How can you increase your light exposure if you exercise indoors? If you exercise at a gym, choose equipment that is located close to a window and face outdoors. Or look for equipment that is located directly under a bank of lights and look at the lights from time to time as you exercise. If you exercise at home, face a window, exercise in the brightest room, or bring extra lights into your workout space. Some people purchase special light boxes that are mounted on stands and place them near their indoor treadmill, stairclimber, or other exercise equipment.

How to Maximize Light Levels Indoors

Breaking Out of the Routine

"BEFORE, I NEVER THOUGHT anything of getting up and going to work in the dark and coming home in the dark. Now I go to the window and I look up at the sky, and I try to get the light in my eyes."

LEVITY volunteer, 33

Once you end your walk or indoor workout, you don't want to be plunged into the gloom. To keep the Body Blues at bay, brighten your interior spaces as well. The older you are, the more important this will be. The lenses of your eyes become more opaque as you age, letting in much less light. For example, an 80-year-old woman needs three times as much light to see as clearly as she did when she was 20. But we should all heed the advice of Cornelius Celsus, a 1st century A.D. Roman savant, who counseled, "live in rooms full of light."

How can you brighten your indoor spaces without sending your electricity bill through the roof? To keep costs down and conserve energy, take advantage of natural daylight as much as possible. Here are some fairly simple and inexpensive strategies.

- Open up the blinds and curtains while you are home and tie them back so they don't block the edges or tops of the windows.

- Consider removing overhanging valances or repositioning them above window height.

- Prune back leggy shrubs and trees that are blocking the light. (Many older homes have "foundation" plantings that have stretched to roof height.)

- Rearrange your furniture so that you can sit close to a window and look outside. (You get at least four times more light when you sit close to a window and look outside as you do when you sit farther away or look away from the window.) If you work at a desk for long hours, it is especially important that you face the outside.

- If you cannot reorient the furniture, place a mirror where it will strategically reflect the outdoor light.

Consider the importance of indoor light as you make long-term plans. For example, if you are hunting for a house or an apartment, search for buildings with large windows, dormers, or skylights. (You'll save on your electricity bill if the windows are double-glazed. The extra pane of glass filters

Does Window Glass Transmit Ultraviolet Light?

Ordinary window glass blocks UVB light, the type long thought to be most damaging to your eyes, but it does allow some UVA light to pass through. In the middle of a room, UVA levels are very low. You are not likely to accumulate hazardous amounts of UVA unless you are sitting with your nose pressed to the window on a sunny day for hours at a time.

Car windows offer substantially more protection than ordinary glass. Clear windshields offer you the same degree of protection as SPF 13 sunscreen, while some tinted car windows with plastic laminates give you an SPF of 500.

out very little additional light.) If you are planning to build a house or have a remodeling budget for your existing home, consider the following tips.

- Brighten rooms by painting the walls and ceilings a light color. Paint with a high-sheen finish bounces around more light than a flatter finish.

- Consider adding dormers, skylights, or sun tubes. (Sun tubes—also called light tubes—are metal cylinders with a reflective inner coating that project through the roof of your house and funnel natural light down into a room. They are less expensive than skylights and easier to install. For more information, see page 163 of the resource section.)

- Think about replacing small windows with larger ones. If your budget allows, purchase windows with a special coating that blocks the UV light and summer heat but traps the warmth during the winter. You can also apply an insulating UV-protective film to existing windows. (There is no universal term for these films. They may be referred to as "solar-protecting," "energy conserving," or "UV-shielding" window films. They can be quite expensive. The films vary in the amount of visible light they transmit. Look for ones that let in the most light.)

- Bring more light into a room by removing a wall and adding windows or glass patio doors.

- Replace an ordinary door with a glass door. (For greater security, use laminated glass or security glass.)

- Think about adding a sunroom—your own daylight spa!
- If you have the resources, consider a home on the water or with a view of the water. Your eyes will be drawn to the view, and you will be rewarded with a double helping of mood-enhancing light.

Boost the Wattage and *Lower* Your Electricity Bill

In addition to bringing more natural light into your house, you can also add more artificial light. The most obvious way is to increase the wattage of your indoor lightbulbs. Some houseware departments even carry 250-watt "reading lights." (Check to see if your lighting fixture can accommodate a higher-watt bulb. The higher the wattage, the more heat the bulb throws off.) If you buy three-way bulbs or install dimmer switches, it will be much easier to have bright light during the day and dim light at night.

The higher the wattage, of course, the more energy you use and the higher your electricity bill. You can compensate for this by turning off lights and appliances when not in use. (Lights equipped with motion detectors do this for you automatically.) But an even better way to save energy is to replace your incandescent bulbs with fluorescent lights. Fluorescent bulbs use about one-quarter as much energy as an incandescent bulb of similar intensity, allowing you to increase your indoor light levels as you *save* money.

Mention the words "fluorescent lights," however, and many people think of the flickering, humming tubes of years gone by that made you look as though you were at death's door. Times have changed. You can now buy new types of fluorescent bulbs that screw into ordinary lighting fixtures and emit a pleasing color with no hum or visible flicker. Called subcompact fluorescents, these high-tech bulbs are an ideal way to relieve the Body Blues but still hold the line on your energy bill. Subcompact fluorescents cost several times more than ordinary bulbs, but you will recoup the cost in less than a year with your energy savings. The bulbs also last much longer than incandescent bulbs (as long as 7 years) and throw off less heat. Look for them in any well-stocked lighting department.

Increased Wattage

"I've increased the wattage in most of my lights. Now, I really, really like well-lit rooms. Before, I always pulled the drapes. I don't like dark rooms at all anymore."

LEVITY volunteer, 42

Purchasing Special Lighting Devices

In our LEVITY study, we helped our volunteers relieve the Body Blues by using natural daylight. But lights designed for phototherapy purposes may be the best option for some people, including older people in retirement facilities and nursing homes, people with physical handicaps that prevent them from getting outdoors, people who can't find time to exercise during the day, and those who prefer to exercise indoors at home.

Light boxes are the most thoroughly tested of all the options. The downside is that they are relatively expensive (from $150 to $450) and anchor you to one place for 30 minutes or more a day. (If you work at a desk, however, you are already tied to one location, so this is not an added inconvenience.) If you want to be mobile and get bright artificial light, consider purchasing a light visor. Light visors are caps equipped with a UV-shielded light that shines directly at your eyes, allowing you freedom of movement. Light visors have been proven to be effective in treating seasonal affective disorder (SAD).[4] Typically, they cost about the same as a light box.

Dawn simulators are yet another option to consider. These are lighting fixtures that you place by the side of your bed and program to turn on early in the morning while you are still sleeping. The light gradually increases in intensity over a period of 45 minutes to an hour, much like the morning sun-

---

Should You Buy Full-Spectrum Lights?

Full-spectrum lights emit a much broader range of radiation than ordinary bulbs, making them more similar in color to sunlight. (To qualify for the designation, lights need to have a color balance that approaches outdoor light at noon.)

Many companies that sell full-spectrum lights advertise them as being the ideal solution for relieving seasonal depression. The lights are indeed effective if they emit 2,500 lux or more. Full-spectrum lights of 150 watts or less, however, do not project enough light to have a no-ticeable effect on your mood.

The jury is still out on whether high-intensity (2,500 lux or more) full-spectrum lights are more effective than white or cool light of equal intensity. Some studies have found that *all* types of light will improve your mood if they are sufficiently bright. Others have given a slight edge to full-spectrum lights. If you wish to purchase full-spectrum lights, look for ones that are UV-shielded. (Some lights that do not have that designation emit a significant amount of ultraviolet radiation.)

light. Eventually, the light is bright enough (100 to 300 lux) to awaken you. Even though the light never reaches the intensity of outdoor light or even a light box, several studies have found them to be as effective in treating SAD as high-intensity light boxes.[5]

Tanning lamps, beds, and booths should *never* take the place of light boxes. In fact, you want to block all the light emitted from tanning equipment from entering your eyes, because it contains UV light. The lamps are shielded to reduce some of the UVB light, which is the part of the spectrum most responsible for sunburns, but it restricts less of the UVA. There is new evidence that UVA light may increase the risk of melanoma, the most deadly type of skin cancer.[6]

Brighten Your Workplace

If have an indoor job, the amount of light in your working environment will have a big impact on how quickly you beat the Body Blues. Factories and large office buildings tend to be more brightly lit than the typical home. You rarely have any control over the light in large buildings, however, and with the growing emphasis on energy conservation and lowering operating costs, many businesses are dimming the light. To maximize your personal light exposure, try to work as close as possible to a window. Alternatively, you can request an additional floor lamp or desk light or bring ones from home. Some people take a portable light box to work and place it close to their work area. Some of the newer devices look like ordinary desk lamps and take up the same amount of space.

Ask your employer about the possibility of painting the walls a lighter color. If you are camped out in a dimly lit cubicle, bring in an extra desk lamp or hang a large mirror on the wall to reflect the light. Suggest that meetings and conferences be held in the sunniest rooms. Take as many outdoor breaks as possible during the day. Eat lunch outdoors or by a window.

There are some very good reasons for your employer to support your efforts to brighten the workplace. A study of 145 office workers found that employees who used a light box for an hour a day in the wintertime felt more vital and had fewer depressive symptoms. This was true whether or not they had the winter blues. The research team concluded that "exposure to bright light may benefit healthy people at large."[7]

What's more, brightening a retail building can have a dramatic effect on sales. A group of consultants surveyed a chain of retail stores to see whether or not sales were influenced by indoor lighting. All the stores had the same design and the same stock of goods. The main difference is that some of the buildings had skylights and others did not. Customers who shopped in the stores with skylights rarely noticed the skylights themselves, but upon questioning, many of them said that the buildings seemed "cleaner" and "more spacious, more open." More important to the chain-store managers, customers also spent a great deal more money. According to this 1999 survey: "All other things being equal, an average non-skylit store in the chain would likely have 40 percent higher sales with the addition of skylights."[8]

Brighten Your Travel

Many people get their greatest light exposure when they are driving their cars. When you are sitting in the driver's seat, you are (1) surrounded by glass, (2) sitting close to the windshield, and (3) looking directly outdoors for sustained periods of time. You can get as much as 1,000 lux of light driving your car on a sunny day. As I explain in "Does Window Glass Transmit Ultraviolet Light?" on page 108, windshields block most of the UV light, so use sunglasses only when needed to reduce the glare. Choose ones with a light tint. If you have a sunroof, open it up whenever conditions allow.

When you travel by bus, train, or plane, choose a window seat. Sit close to a window when you ride in a cab. If you're stuck at an airport waiting for a plane, sit near a large window and face outside. While you're waiting for a ride, stand outside rather than inside, weather permitting. If you walk, bike, skate, or ride a scooter to work, you are already getting the full dose of light plus exercise as well—congratulations!

When you take a vacation, consider going to a sunny location. If you can plan a sun break in the middle of winter, you will reduce your risk of winter depression. If you are retired and live in a northern state, consider joining the "snowbirds" and migrating to the South when it gets dark and gloomy at home. A trip to snowy areas also enhances your light exposure. (When you are vacationing in a very bright area, however, it will be especially important to protect your eyes and your skin from UV light.)

Let There Be Dark

Until the 20th century, people were exposed to very little light after sunset. Now, with the flip of a switch, we can illuminate the night. But too much light late at night sends a confusing message to our bodies' hormonal command center: Is it night? Is it day? Is it time to get up or go to bed?

When night falls, your body "expects" to be in the dark. As discussed earlier, one of the consequences of getting bright light at night is that your melatonin production is delayed or blunted. Abnormal melatonin levels have been linked with a number of psychiatric disorders, including SAD, bipolar disorder (formerly known as manic-depression), unipolar depression, bulimia, anorexia, schizophrenia, panic disorder, and obsessive-compulsive disorder.[9]

To make sure that you are not compromising your nighttime supply of melatonin, turn down the lights at night. If you read at night, use only enough light to see what's on the page. If your partner keeps the lights on in the bedroom when you want to sleep, wear a light-blocking sleep mask or sleep in another room. Install dimmer switches in the bathroom and bedroom so that you can have bright light in the morning and soothing, dim light at night. If city lights come in your windows at night, install light-blocking shades or, again, wear a sleep mask.

When you have succeeded in creating a more natural lighting environment, your body will be back in sync with the sun. You will feel more energized during the daytime and sleep more soundly at night. You will have fewer food cravings and feel less compelled to overeat. As was true for many of our LEVITY volunteers, this environmental change may seem so beneficial to you that within weeks it no longer feels like a "program requirement" but a better and more natural way to live.

Questions and Answers

Q. How can I determine how much light is in my indoor environment, both at work and at home?

A. The best way to find out is to borrow or purchase a device called a lux meter, which is available through your local camera shop. (You can also visit www.thebodyblues.com for specific recommendations.) Explain that you are looking for a handheld light meter that measures light in a range from 25 to 50,000 lux. Some light meters measure in foot-candles (fc), which is fine, but you will need to convert lux into foot-candles to make sense of the information in this book. (To convert lux into foot-candles, multiply lux times 0.0929. For example, 1,000 lux multiplied by 0.0929 equals approximately 92.9 foot-candles. To convert foot-candles into lux, multiply by 10.76. For example, 92.9 foot-candles multiplied by 10.76 equals approximately 1,000 lux.)

Q. Can I get too much light during the daytime?

A. You can certainly get too much *UV* light, so do what you can to cut down your exposure. There is no known hazard from getting too much outdoor light in the visible (non-UV) spectrum, however—other than eye fatigue from glare.

Yet a minority of people do have mild adverse reactions to light boxes. Some have visual complaints, although no significant eye damage has been reported. Some feel overstimulated, jittery, or agitated. Headaches are rare, but not unknown. Spending less time in front of the light, using it less often, or switching to a dimmer light fixture can solve all of these problems. People with bipolar disorder should use phototherapy devices only under the supervision of their mental health specialist, because too much light can trigger a manic episode.[10]

Q. I work the night shift, so I rarely can take a walk in the daylight hours. What can I do to elevate my mood?

A. One in five Americans now works the night shift, and the number is expected to rise as demand increases for round-the-clock production and service. The best time to get bright light is at the beginning of your subjective workday, because it will shut off melatonin production and stimulate activating chemicals. If possible, get up early enough to spend 20 minutes outside before the sun sets. If you can't, consider purchasing a bright artificial light and using it 30 minutes each day right before you go to work.

Q. I'm a landscape designer and spend several hours outside each day. I think I get plenty of light as it is. Do I still need to get more light?

A. Probably not. Studies suggest that for normal functioning, you need to get at least 1,000 lux of light for 1 hour a day. You are getting that much light and more on your job. You might try bringing more light into your home, however, and see if it makes any improvement in your symptoms. If you see no change, there's no need to go to the trouble (unless other family members are showing signs of light deprivation).

Q. My 12-year-old daughter seems to get depressed in the winter. Her grades slip. She stays by herself much of the time. She's less cooperative. All this goes away in the spring. Will bright lights help her?

A. Most children and adolescents have a dip in mood in the winter, just like adults. If the symptoms are pronounced, getting more light can relieve them. I suggest you discuss the matter with your daughter's health care provider to rule out other causes of low mood.

Q. Does it matter how much light my children are getting at school?

A. A 1999 survey of more than 21,000 children living in California, Washington, and Colorado compared the amount of light in the children's classrooms with their reading and math scores. Although the various school districts had different curricula, teaching styles, building designs, and climates, the children in rooms with the most daylight consistently scored higher on tests of math and reading than children in rooms with the least daylight. In the school district that provided the most complete data, the students in the rooms with the most daylight "progressed 20 percent faster on math tests and 26 percent faster on reading tests in 1 year than those with the least [daylight]." The investigators concluded that "by advancing more quickly, students in daylit classrooms could save up to 1 month of instruction time in the reading and math curriculum that could be used for other areas of learning."[11] School teachers and administrators, take note.

Q. My mother lives in a nursing home. Will brightening her indoor environment improve her mood?

A. Bright light is especially important for older people because their eyes do not absorb as much light and because they tend to spend much less time outdoors than younger people. (One study found that the healthy elderly get one-third the amount of light exposure as younger people. Alzheimer's patients get even less, and women with Alzheimer's get the least light of all.)[12]

Talk to your older family members or friends about increasing the amount of light in their homes. Suggest installing subcompact fluorescents to keep the energy bill down. If a parent is living in a nursing home or assisted-living facility, see if he or she can be moved to a sunnier room or have a bed by the window. Bring in lighting fixtures and brighter bulbs. Install large mirrors to bounce the light around the room. Make sure the blinds are open in the daytime. Many assisted-living facilities have sunrooms or covered patio areas. The more time your parent spends in these bright areas, the better. If you have a parent with Alzheimer's disease, bright light may improve his or her sleep and even relieve agitation in the late afternoon and early evening.[13]

Your Turn

The following exercises will help you develop your own plan for bringing more light into your environment. They will also aid in identifying and eliminating potential stumbling blocks.

Exercise 1. Making Plans to Improve Your Lighting Environment

In this chapter, I've discussed a number of ways to create a more natural lighting environment. Look at the list below and check the ones that seem most helpful and practical for you. Then put an X beside those that you plan to act upon within a week.

By next week, I plan to . . .

____ Go for outdoor walks five or more times a week.

____ Look straight ahead or at the sky while walking on darker days.

____ Walk near a body of water (when possible) on darker days.

____ Use a transparent umbrella when it rains or snows.

____ Wear lightly tinted or clear sunglasses for UV protection.

____ Have a special UV coating applied to my prescription glasses.

____ Switch to UV-shielded contacts.

____ Eat a diet rich in antioxidants and other eye-protecting nutrients.

____ Open blinds and curtains in the daytime.

____ Remove overhanging valances.

____ Prune trees and shrubs that are preventing the light from entering the house.

____ Rearrange some furniture to face toward the windows.

____ Place large mirrors to reflect more light.

____ Paint walls a brighter color.

____ Add sun tubes, skylights, or dormers.

____ Add windows, glass doors, or a sunroom.

____ Install brighter lightbulbs in strategic locations indoors.

____ Switch to subcompact fluorescent bulbs.

____ Rearrange work furniture.

____ Bring lighting fixtures, brighter bulbs, or a light box to work.

____ Choose window seats on public transportation whenever possible.

____ Plan a winter vacation in a sunny location.

____ Purchase a light box, light visor, or dawn simulator.

____ Turn down indoor lights in the late evening.

____ Install dimmer switches in bathrooms and bedrooms.

____ Wear a sleep mask at night.

____ Install light-blocking shades in the bedroom.

____ Other: _____

_____

_____

_____

Exercise 2. Overcoming Obstacles

Can you foresee any problems you might have in creating brighter days and darker nights? If so, what are they?

_____

_____

_____

_____

_____

_____

_____

_____

What are some ways to resolve these problems? (Brainstorm with friends and family members if you need to come up with more alternatives.)

_____

_____

_____

_____

_____

_____

_____

_____

Chapter 8

Walk Away
from Your Body Blues

Getting the Most from Your 20-Minute Walks

In this chapter, I'll be giving you detailed instructions and helpful hints for the second LEVITY activity: getting 20 minutes of moderate-intensity exercise. Most of my comments will be about brisk outdoor walking, but other activities will also satisfy the exercise component of the program. For example, if you prefer, you can spend your 20 minutes snowshoeing, cross-country skiing, skating, hiking, biking, kayaking, stairclimbing, dancing, or rowing. You can also switch from one activity to another as the spirit moves you. I encourage you to choose any type of exercise you wish, as long as it meets the following criteria:

1. You enjoy it.
2. You stay within the "feel-good" zone, which means exercising fast enough to stimulate your mind and body but not so fast that you feel out of breath or stressed.
3. You exercise five or more times a week for 20 minutes or more.
4. You exercise outdoors or find some other way to get 20 minutes of bright light (1,000 lux or more) each day.

Defining the Feel-Good Zone

Whether you choose walking or some other activity, your goal is to exercise at about 60 percent of your maximum heart rate (MHR). This is the rate that has been found to be ideal for elevating mood, lowering stress and anxiety, and stimulating the production of appetite-suppressing chemicals. There is a simple formula for calculating 60 percent of your MHR. Take the number

60 Percent of Maximum Heart Rate

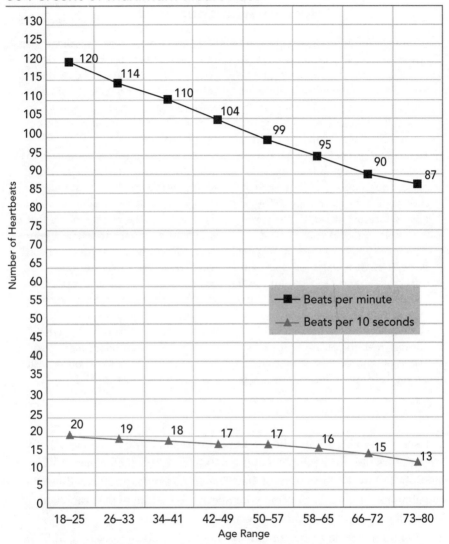

To determine 60 percent of your maximum heart rate, first locate your age range at the bottom of the graph. Draw a line straight up from your age range so that it intersects the two lines on the graph. The bottom line tells you the number of beats per 10 seconds. The top line tells you approximately how many times your heart should be beating in 60 seconds.

As an example, if you are 40 years old, draw a line up from the 34–41 range until it meets the two lines on the graph. If you are counting your pulse for 10 seconds, your heart should be beating approximately 18 times. If you are counting it for a full minute, it should be beating about 110 times. If it's beating much slower or faster, adjust your speed accordingly.

How to Take Your Pulse

If you've never taken your own pulse before, first practice while sitting still. Place two fingers of one hand on the underside of your wrist, straight down from your index finger. If you can't feel your pulse, move your fingers until you find it. The carotid artery in your neck is another place to try. To find this artery, place your fingers on the side of your neck close to your jaw. (The artery is located straight down from the outer corner of your eye.)

Once you have located your pulse, look at a watch or clock with a second hand and count your heartbeats for 10 seconds. Multiply that number by 6 to give you the number of beats per minute. (A normal resting pulse ranges between 60 and 80 beats per minute, although some athletes have a rate of 50 or less. Certain medications can also speed up or slow down your pulse.) Once you have taken your pulse sitting down, practice while walking. (You may have to stop a moment to be able to detect your heartbeat.)

A few people find it difficult to take their own pulse, especially while exercising. If this is true for you, consider purchasing a heart rate monitor. There are models that attach to a finger, go around your wrist, or strap around your chest. You can even purchase one that gives you an audible readout of your heart rate, elapsed time, how many calories you've burned, and how much distance you've traveled. (For more information, see page 167 of the resource section or visit www.thebodyblues.com.)

220, subtract your age, and then multiply the result by 60 percent (0.6). If you are 40 years old, for example, subtract 40 from 220, which equals 180. Then multiply 180 by 0.6 for a total of 108. The graph on page 119 has done these calculations for you. Simply find your age at the bottom of the graph and then locate the appropriate number directly above.

You do not need to be compulsive about exercising precisely at 60 percent of your MHR, however. Aim to keep within 5 beats or so. If your target number is 108, for example, aim to stay within 103 to 113 heartbeats per minute. If you fall below this range, pick up the pace. If you climb above, slow it down. After checking your pulse frequently during several walks, you will develop a good sense of how fast you need to go without having to check.

How quickly you will need to walk to stay in the ideal zone varies greatly from person to person. This was very evident to us as we were helping our LEVITY volunteers find the right pace during their orientation sessions. Even though all the women were walking at 60 percent of their MHR, some appeared to be going for a leisurely stroll while others looked like competitors in a racewalk. One reason for the variability in speed is that a person's MHR declines with age, so the older women were aiming for a lower pulse rate. For example, a 20-year-old woman will be aiming for a pulse rate of about 120 beats per minute while a 70-year-old will be striving for only 90 beats a minute.

Another reason for the different walking speeds was variation in physical fitness and body weight. The women who were the most fit had more efficient hearts and lower resting pulse rates. As a consequence, they had to walk considerably faster to reach 60 percent of their MHR. (I have been exercising for years, so I have a very low resting pulse rate. To reach 60 percent of my MHR, I have to jog.) Women who were heavier or less fit had higher resting pulse rates and therefore could achieve their goal at a much slower speed. The only way to know how fast *you* need to walk is by taking your pulse the first few times you exercise.

If you have been living a very sedentary lifestyle, in just a few weeks you will be more fit and have a lower resting heart rate. To keep your heart beating within the desired range, you will have to walk more quickly, pump your arms more vigorously, or add a hill to your walk. Fortunately, your walks won't seem any more strenuous than they did in the beginning, because you will have increased stamina. (Note: If you are 60 or older, have a known physical problem, or have been very inactive in the past few months, take the quick test on page 131 before you begin walking. Called the Physical Activity Readiness Questionnaire, or PAR-Q, it will tell you whether you need your practitioner's approval before starting the exercise portion of the LEVITY program.)

How Often and How Long Should You Exercise?

Exercising for 20 minutes a day, 5 days a week is enough physical activity to relieve the Body Blues. If you want to exercise more, so much the better. You'll be burning more calories, creating firmer muscles, and enjoying more of the short-term benefits of exercise. Just make sure that a longer session or walking more frequently doesn't make you feel stressed. The goal is to make exercise an enjoyable, stress-*reducing* part of your day.

On days when you can't squeeze in the full 20 minutes, I recommend that you walk for as many minutes as possible, even if it's only a turn around the block. In a study published in 2000, volunteers who walked for just 10 to 15 minutes felt more energetic during the walk and felt calmer and more relaxed afterward.[1] Even walking for as little as 5 minutes will help sustain your momentum. It will be easier to go back to the full 20 minutes when you've been walking a few minutes a day than when you've slipped back into a completely sedentary mode.

Posture Perfect

You already know how to walk, of course, but if you concentrate on having good posture, you will reduce the tension in your shoulders and tone your upper torso as well. The most important piece of advice is to think "tall" as you walk. Imagine that there is a string attached to the top of your head, which is pulling you up and elongating your spine. Pull up your rib cage so that you increase the distance between the bottom of your ribs and your waist. Pull in your stomach as you walk so that you will be toning your abdominal muscles and relieving the strain on your back. Tuck your pelvis slightly down and under. A slightly tucked pelvis will prevent you from walking with a sway back. (To get a sense of the proper alignment, stand with your back and shoulders against a wall and then place a hand on the small of your back. Tilt your pelvis under until your hand is snug against the wall.) As you walk, keep your head level and your shoulders down, square, and relaxed. Every 5 minutes or so, stop and roll your neck and shoulders.

As you walk, lean slightly forward from your ankles, but not from your waist. (If you lean forward from your waist, you will be putting strain on your back and making it more difficult to breathe.) Walk with a stride length that is only slightly longer than usual. If you need to walk faster, move more quickly rather than lengthening your stride. Push off with your back foot and land on the heel of your front foot, rolling smoothly from your heel through your arch to your toes. Push off with your toes.

Pump your arms. How fast you pump them will help regulate your heart rate. Pump more vigorously if you're below the desired range; move them in a smaller arc if your heart rate is too fast. If you have to carry something on your walk, put it in a cart, backpack, or fanny pack

Midday Break

"I FOUND THAT GOING for walks in the middle of my workday lets me just walk away from my annoying coworker and just go—walk away and get that break. It made me realize how good that made me feel. It was like exerting my own power kind of thing."

LEVITY volunteer, 25

so you can balance the load and free up your arms. Finally—remember to look straight ahead or glance up at the sky occasionally so that you get your full quota of energizing, mood-elevating light!

Choosing the Right Shoes and Socks

> ### Always Ready to Walk
>
> "I KEEP A PAIR of walking shoes and a rain parka in my car so that I can take advantage of odd moments—like waiting for my daughters to get out of school or finish their music lessons."
>
> **LEVITY volunteer, 30**

The most essential piece of equipment you will need on your walk is a comfortable, supportive pair of walking shoes. You will be logging a lot of miles—400 to 600 miles each year. Make sure that your shoes fit and are well-suited for the purpose. Shoes designed especially for walking have extra cushioning at the heel and ball of the foot to absorb shock. (The heavier and older you are, the more important this padding will be. The natural padding at the bottom of your foot thins with age.) The heels of the shoes are slightly rounded (rather than the squared-off heel typical of a running shoe) to encourage you to roll evenly from your heel to your toes. The shoes are flexible at the toes, but not the arch.

For advice on what brand of walking shoe to buy, look for a review in *Consumer Reports*, a sports and fitness magazine, or a Web site devoted to walking. Even more important, make sure that the shoes are well-designed for your particular feet. Shoes are constructed on wooden or composite forms called lasts, which vary from manufacturer to manufacturer and model to model. Parts that vary the most are the heel width, width at the ball of the foot, height of the toebox, and height of the arch. To know what suits you best, go to a store with a wide selection of shoes and trained personnel who specialize in assuring the correct fit.

If you have a tendency to walk on the inside or outside of your feet (over- or underpronate) ask for *motion-control* or *stability* shoes that help align your feet in the proper position. If you have knee or foot pain when you start walking, consult a podiatrist. These foot specialists can solve many problems by designing custom inserts (orthotics) or simply by giving specific advice on what style and brand of shoe to wear.

Even the best shoes will wear out over time, diminishing their support and cushioning properties. Plan on buying a new pair at least once a year. If you will be walking in the rain a great deal, buy two pairs so one pair can dry out while you wear the other. (Stuff wads of newspaper in the shoes so they will keep their shape as they dry. Keep them away from sunlight and heat.) If you live in an area with lots of snow, you can (1) buy walking shoes with extra traction, (2) invest in a pair of the newer lightweight snowshoes, (3) buy strap-on snow or ice treads, or (4) use rubber "slip-ons" with steel cleats.

If you're going for a 20-minute walk on a dry day with no extremes in temperature, you can wear any pair of socks that happens to be at the top of the drawer as long as the socks fit comfortably and don't bunch up at the heel. But if it's a wet, cold, or hot day, avoid cotton socks because they can become cold and clammy or hot and sweaty within minutes. Instead, wear socks or sock liners made from synthetic fibers, such as acrylic or DuPont's CoolMax, that wick moisture away from your skin. If your feet are dry, you will feel more comfortable and be less likely to have problems with blisters.

Weatherproofing

In inclement conditions, pay attention to the rest of your clothing as well. Finding the time to squeeze in regular walks is enough of a challenge that you don't want to have to cope with feeling cold, clammy, sweaty, or wet.

In some parts of the country and times of the year, heat is the biggest concern. The best time of day to exercise during hot weather is early in the morning when the air is coolest and the UV index is low. (UV peaks from 10:00 A.M. to 2:00 P.M.) The most comfortable clothes to wear on a very hot day are light-colored mesh tank tops and loose-fitting shorts, both made from synthetic material. Your undergarments should be made from synthetic, wicking material as well. (There are companies that specialize in no-nonsense sportswear for women. Look for links at www.thebodyblues.com.) Protect your bare skin with sunscreen. If you want to be more covered up, wear loose-fitting acrylic tops and pants. A ventilated hat with a broad brim will keep the sun from beating down on your head. Low-cut shoes and socks will help reduce heat buildup.

Just as important as choosing the right clothes is staying hydrated. Drink water *before*, during, and after your exercise session to stave off dehydration. Carry a water

---

Keeps Clothing Together

"I HAD TO CONSCIOUSLY make sure that I had my clothing thing together. I hate to be cold, so I bought a warm fleece jacket, hat, and gloves. I keep the hat and gloves in the pocket so I don't have to search for them."

LEVITY volunteer, 36

bottle. In addition to drinking the water, you can douse your head, face, and neck. Or carry a spritz bottle to mist your face. (This is especially helpful for women who are slow to sweat.)

During a heat wave, either go for your walk as soon as the sun comes up or exercise in an air-conditioned gym, in a shopping mall, or at home. Thousands of shopping malls open their doors early in the morning just for walkers, and some even have organized walking groups.

Enjoying the Rain

"I KNOW IT'S A FUNNY thing to say, but I find I really look forward to walking in the rain. Everybody else is inside, so I have the park all to myself. People think they melt in the rain, but you don't. You just have to have the right gear. When I open my see-through umbrella, I feel like I'm in a protective bubble."

LEVITY volunteer, 29

Layering is the solution for cold, wet, or windy days. Think of your clothing as having three layers: (1) an inner, wicking layer; (2) a middle, insulating layer; and (3) an outer layer to repel the wind, rain, or snow. The innermost layer, including your undergarments, should be made from a wickable, synthetic fabric as discussed earlier. Depending on the temperature, this inner layer can be anything from a silky, lightweight top to polypropylene long johns. The second, insulating layer can range from a T-shirt to polar fleece. (There is a new type of polar fleece called Windbloc, produced by Malden Mills, that is designed to shield you from the wind.) If conditions are dry and calm, you may be able to dispense with an outer layer. But on rainy, windy, or snowy days, wear a breathable water-resistant jacket made from Gore-Tex or similar material or a loose-fitting, rubberized slicker. (A slicker is not appropriate for long walks or more strenuous exercise because it does not allow moisture to evaporate.) As soon as your body begins to heat up, unzip the outer layer or shed an insulating layer. You will feel more energized if you don't get too warm.

On the coldest days, wear mittens rather than gloves. (Glove liners specifically designed to trap body heat are great on bitterly cold days and for people with Raynaud's phenomenon, a condition in which blood vessels constrict abnormally in stressful or cold conditions.) Wear a warm hat that covers your head and ears. If conditions are extremely cold or icy, exercise indoors. (One of the volunteers in our study walked in place on her covered deck whenever it was pouring down rain. This would also work on icy days.)

Exercising Indoors

A few women in our study found it inconvenient to exercise outdoors. They had too little free time during daylight hours, greatly preferred exercising indoors, or were too unstable on their feet to walk unassisted. During the orientation session, we helped them identify ways to get more light indoors while they exercised. Some women moved their exercise equipment so that it faced a window. Others turned on very bright lights. One woman used a portable light box, and another relied on a light visor.

Some women chose to get their light and exercise at separate times. For example, a woman who wore a suit and heels to work and often had 30 minutes for lunch found it impractical to change clothes and go for a walk in that brief amount of time. She decided to eat lunch outside whenever possible or eat lunch while looking out her window. On her way home from work, she stopped and exercised at the gym. For every situation, there is a solution.

Make Exercise a Priority

If you exercise for less than 20 minutes a day, 5 days a week, your benefits will decrease. If you slip below 3 days a week on a regular basis, it's time to do some problem solving. First, identify what is keeping you from exercising. (Exercise 4 on page 135 is designed to do just that.) If you are chronically "too busy" to exercise—the most common reason—examine your priorities. Twenty minutes is only $\frac{1}{48}$ of your waking day. That's very little time to set aside for an activity that gives you so many proven benefits.

Many of the women I see in my practice place their work responsibilities and/or the needs of their friends and family members above their own. Society colludes by rewarding them for being good workers, moms, friends, daughters, or partners—but *not* for spending a half-hour a day restoring their energy and spirits. The net result is that they feel so depleted that they underperform at work and disappoint the people they care about most.

If you have a tendency to shortchange yourself, think about the advice airline attendants give at the beginning of a flight: "If oxygen masks should appear, put on your own mask before helping others." Clearly, you are of little use to other passengers if you are gasping for oxygen. This is a good analogy for life in general. You need to take care of yourself first. If you don't, you run the risk of being ill, doing poorly at work, being an impatient parent, or neglecting family and friends. Think of your 20-minute walk as your private time, your opportunity to recharge your batteries. Ultimately, taking regular walks will benefit all the people and causes you care about, as well as yourself.

Motivate Yourself

The best form of self-motivation is pleasure. When you enjoy what you're doing, the motivation flows effortlessly. For this reason, I encourage you to think of all the ways that you can make your walks more pleasurable. If you enjoy nature, scout out walking trails in parks and other beautiful locations. (Call your local parks and recreation department for information.) If your schedule has little room for socializing, walk with a friend, partner, or a group of friends. If you walk by yourself, consider using the time for contemplation and problem solving—or entertain yourself with music or books on tape. If you like your walks to have a purpose, walk to a favorite destination. Exercise 2 on page 133 gives you an A-to-Z list of suggestions that will help make your walks an oasis of calm and pleasure.

But as everyone knows, it's possible to stop doing something that you really enjoy if circumstances intervene. You look back in time and think, "I used to love doing that. How come I don't do it anymore?" For some women, a good way to stay on track is to keep careful records. We gave logbooks to our study volunteers so they could record how often and how long they walked. Some found the record keeping a chore and did it only because we asked them to. But others found the exercise very helpful. "I don't want to have a blank day in the logbook," reported a 19-year-old University of Washington student. "I feel so virtuous making all those checks." A second woman told us that having a history of her walks helped her get going again after having the flu. "I looked back at all those checks and saw that I had been very faithful to the program for 3 weeks. Somehow, that made it easier for me to start again. I didn't feel I was starting from scratch. I was simply picking up where I left off." If you think you would benefit from keeping a journal, you'll find sample pages on page 154 of this book that you can photocopy for your own use.

Library of Audiotapes

"I DISCOVERED THAT my library has audiotapes of some of my favorite romance novels. So I made a bargain with myself that I would listen to them only during my walks. Sometimes I can hardly wait for the next walk to hear more of the story. And often I'll keep on walking longer than 20 minutes just to get to the end of a chapter."

LEVITY volunteer, 51

Walking Brought Calm

"LAST SATURDAY I WAS FEELING so resentful of my family I felt like screaming. Instead, I told my husband I was going for a walk and that he'd have to take over. An interesting thing happened during my walk. At first, I was fuming. Then about 10 minutes into the walk, a feeling of calm gradually came over me. Then, without even trying, I began to have these positive feelings about my husband. When I came back a half-hour later, I was fit to live with again. I stayed sane all day."

LEVITY volunteer, 28

Advice for the Reluctant Walker

Do you have doubts that you will be able to motivate yourself to go for frequent walks? The good news is that the more sedentary you are, the more you will benefit physically and mentally from exercise. But first, you need to overcome your inertia. Learning about the mood benefits of exercise has probably given you some incentive to get moving. But don't count on a spontaneous urge to exercise to get you out the door. If you had the inclination to be physically active, you'd be doing so already. *To begin the program, you may have to go for walks even though you don't want to.*

It might help to start out gradually. The first time you walk, for example, just go around the block. Each day, add a few more minutes. As you wait for walking to become an ingrained habit, rely on external rewards. For example, the first week that you walk three times at the recommended pace, reward yourself in some special way such as getting an hour-long massage, hiring a babysitter and going to a movie, or taking a personal day off from work. Or buy something that gives you pleasure. (I love to buy gear and gadgets when I start something new. When I started kayaking, for example, I suited myself out with all the appropriate gear.)

Gadgets that go along with a walking program include a heart rate monitor to keep track of your pulse, a pedometer to record your distance, a portable CD player, new exercise clothes, all-weather gear, water bottles and water bottle holsters, visors, a fanny pack or backpack, and a transparent umbrella for rainy days. Eventually, you will be getting so much intrinsic reward from your walks that you can let go of some of the external inducements.

Questions and Answers

Q. How much weight will I lose by walking five times a week?

A. How quickly you lose weight is influenced by your activity level, age, genetics, current weight, and, of course, the number of calories you consume. A woman of average size burns about 150 calories during each 20-minute walk. If you walk five times a week, that amounts to about 750 extra calories per week, which translates into about a pound weight loss each month, or 11 to 12 pounds per year. Clearly, going for short walks is not a "Lose 20 Pounds Overnight" miracle cure. To lose weight more quickly, exercise for longer periods of time and reduce your caloric intake by about 500 calories a day.

A Forced Time-Out

"BEFORE THE STUDY, I was in this slump where I almost couldn't go outside. The program forced me to get out. I started walking during my morning break. And then it felt so good, I decided to do it on my afternoon break, too. It helped me think about what was bothering me. It was like my little exercise to identify what the problems were and decide what to do about them. Sometimes, I would go home from work and want to go for a walk after work, too."

LEVITY volunteer, 37

Q. Do I need to add a warmup and cooldown period to my 20-minute exercise session?

A. Your level of exertion will be moderate enough that you probably won't need either one. But it will help to stretch *after* your walk. (It's best to stretch when your muscles are warm.) Stretching will help keep you limber and supple.

Q. I like to run. Can I jog for 20 minutes instead of walk?

A. Unless you are in very good physical condition, jogging will increase your heart rate above 60 percent of your maximum heart rate. That is fine, however, if you can jog or run without feeling stressed or fatigued. For some very fit people, a jog *feels* like a walk.

Q. Can I vary the type of physical activity from day to day?

A. Indeed you can. For many women, this is the best way to keep from becoming bored with an exercise program. When you switch from one activity to another, you also exercise more muscle groups. Take your pulse at least once during each new type of physical activity so you can determine if you are exercising at the right pace.

Q. I like to walk with friends, but I don't think they will keep up the pace. What should I do?

A. Perhaps you can convince some of your friends to go on the LEVITY program with you. Then you will all be motivated to walk at a brisk pace. You can saunter with your more laid-back friends at other times.

Q. I like to walk with my boyfriend, but he has long legs and walks much faster than I do. I have to jog to keep up. Is this a problem?

A. It *is* a problem if you feel uncomfortable walking that fast and feel pressured to keep up. Have your boyfriend read chapter 5 of this book so that he understands the importance of exercising within your comfort zone. If he finds it too difficult to slow down, he can jog a few blocks ahead of you and then circle back while you keep at a steady pace.

Q. If I exercise during my lunch break at work, there's no opportunity to shower when I get back. I also don't like to sweat in general. This is one of the things that has kept me from exercising in the past. Any suggestions?

A. If you wear appropriate clothing, there's no need to work up a sweat during a 20-minute walk. First, make a practice of wearing a bra and panties made from a wicking, synthetic material. (You will find these at women's athletic apparel stores or on the Internet. You will enjoy the added comfort even on those days when you don't go for a walk. Some fabrics have even been treated to prevent the growth of odor-causing bacteria.) Before going for your walk, take off your work clothes and slip on a weather-appropriate middle layer, which could be anything from a mesh tank top to polar fleece. If it's cold and rainy, add a breathable shell that will keep you dry but allow moisture to evaporate. *As soon as your body starts to heat up, unzip your jacket or start shedding layers.* Don't let the heat build up unnecessarily.

Q. I'm more than 100 pounds overweight and haven't been able to walk for more than 5 minutes for years. How can I participate in the exercise part of the LEVITY program?

A. There are many women in your situation. Before going for your first walk, check with your primary care provider to see if there is any reason that you should not take part in a program of moderate-intensity exercise. (In addition, take the test on the next page. The PAR-Q is a quick test of exercise readiness, but it does not take the place of seeing a practitioner.) Once you get the go-ahead, begin gradually. Walk for 3 minutes at any pace the first day. If you feel fine during and after the walk, go for 3 minutes the next day as well. Add more minutes as your degree of physical fitness allows. One test of your readiness to increase your walk is being able to talk without being short of breath.

If walking seems too ambitious or if you'd prefer to exercise inside, consider buying an exercise video specially designed for overweight people.

How Fit Are You?

If you have been sedentary in the past few months or have a known medical condition, take this simple test before beginning the exercise component of the LEVITY program.

THE "PAR-Q" (Physical Activity Readiness Questionnaire)[2]

Instructions: Place a check mark by the appropriate answer to each of the following seven questions.

1. Has a doctor ever said that you have a heart condition and recommended only medically supervised activity?
   Yes ☐ No ☐

2. Do you have chest pain brought on by physical activity?
   Yes ☐ No ☐

3. Have you developed chest pain in the past month?
   Yes ☐ No ☐

4. Do you tend to lose consciousness or fall as a result of dizziness?
   Yes ☐ No ☐

5. Do you have a bone or joint problem that could be aggravated by the proposed physical activity?
   Yes ☐ No ☐

6. Has a doctor ever recommended medication for your blood pressure or a heart condition?
   Yes ☐ No ☐

7. Are you aware, through your own experience or a doctor's advice, of any other physical reason against your exercising without medical supervision?
   Yes ☐ No ☐

If you accurately and honestly answered no to all questions, you have reasonable assurance that you are fit enough to begin exercising. If you answered yes to one or more questions, postpone this part of the program until you get medical consultation and clearance.

Note: There is *no* guarantee that any protection from sudden death is afforded by *any* pretest, even those more complex than PAR-Q.

(Visit www.thebodyblues.com for recommendations.) Some videos feature chair exercises that you perform sitting down. Turn on very bright lights as you exercise so that you benefit from light therapy as well. (Remember that light alone can help you lose weight.)

Pay special attention to your shoes. Make sure that they fit well and offer sufficient support. You may need custom orthotics (shoe inserts) or even custom-made shoes. If you get your health care provider to prescribe them, your insurance may cover or offset the expense.

Your Turn

The exercises below will help you clarify your reasons for exercising, identify ways to make your walks more enjoyable, and develop a plan to overcome known difficulties.

Exercise 1. What Are Your Reasons for Exercising?

It's human nature to weigh the costs and benefits of any activity. This first exercise will help you focus on the benefits of being more active. The greater your perceived benefits, the more likely you are to follow through.

Directions: Below is a list of some of the proven rewards of moderate-intensity exercise, including mood and health benefits. Check the ones that are important to you. Then go back and underline the three that have the most meaning for you. Write those three benefits on a card or piece of paper and place it where you will see it every day.

❏ Less stress
❏ Less anxiety
❏ More energy
❏ Decreased appetite
❏ A more positive mood
❏ Gradual weight loss
❏ Better posture
❏ Improved cardiovascular fitness
❏ A lower risk of diabetes
❏ Lower LDL (bad) cholesterol levels
❏ Higher HDL (good) cholesterol levels
❏ A lower risk of cancer
❏ Toned muscles
❏ Increased strength
❏ Better balance
❏ Restored faith in the ability to stick with an exercise program
❏ Taking personal responsibility for solving the Body Blues

❐ Being a role model for family or friends
❐ Better sleep at night
❐ Other: _____

_____

_____

Exercise 2. What Makes Exercise Pleasurable for You?

Part of your responsibility in the LEVITY program is to find ways to make your walking or other moderate-intensity exercise as pleasurable as possible. Ideally, you want to look forward to your 20-minute session. This exercise gives you some suggestions.

Directions: Circle the letters of the ideas that seem most appealing to you. Add at least one idea to the blank space at the end of the list. Then go back and highlight the ones that spark your interest the most.

I will enjoy exercising more if I . . .

a. Exercise by myself so I can be free of the demands of other people and think my own thoughts.
b. Exercise with a partner, friend, or child.
c. Exercise with a group of friends.
d. Walk in a shopping mall.
e. Listen to my favorite music.
f. Listen to educational or work-related tapes.
g. Listen to inspirational tapes.
h. Listen to books on audiotapes.
i. Walk in a beautiful setting.
j. Use a pedometer or heart rate monitor.
k. Have a particular destination such as a friend's house or a local store.
l. Go somewhere that I can engage in "people watching."
m. Walk along favorite urban streets.
n. Vary where I walk.
o. Stick to the same path.
p. Use the time to focus on all that I'm grateful for.
q. Use the time to solve personal or work difficulties.
r. Walk a dog.
s. Discover new parts of the city.
t. Learn more about nature.
u. Take binoculars along.

v. Take a camera along.

w. Create my own walking tape or CD.

x. Take along a tape recorder to record my thoughts, make lists, or dictate work-related matters.

y. Come home and treat myself to a favorite ritual such as drinking a hot cup of tea and reading the paper, or taking a soak in the tub.

z. Switch from one type of exercise to another.

Other: _____

_____

_____

Exercise 3. Putting Your Plan into Action

It's one thing to identify what would make your exercise more pleasing to you; it's another to put it into action. This third exercise will help you realize your ideas.

Directions: In the space provided below, list several of the activities that will make your exercise session more appealing to you. Then write down how you plan to put them into action.

EXAMPLE:

Idea: *I would like to walk with a group of friends from my church.*

Action Plan: *I will share this book with my friends and see who's interested in joining a walking group. Then I will invite the ones who are interested to my house to work out a schedule.*

Idea: _____

_____

Action Plan: _____

_____

_____

Idea: _____

_____

Action Plan: _____

_____

_____

Idea: _____

_____

Action Plan: _____

_____

_____

Exercise 4. Overcoming Obstacles

Have you started exercise programs before and had trouble sticking with them? You will find the LEVITY program easier to maintain than most because it requires only a moderate amount of exertion. Nonetheless, it helps to identify obstacles that have tripped you up in the past so that you can avoid them this time around.

Directions: Below are some of the most common reasons for not exercising. (There is a space to add additional items at the bottom.) Put an X by those factors that have sabotaged your good intentions in the past.

_____ Not setting aside enough time to exercise

_____ Problems with child care

_____ Fatigue

_____ Lack of support from others

_____ Boredom

_____ Injuries

_____ Fear of injury

_____ Not knowing all the benefits of exercise

_____ A history of failure with exercise programs

_____ Setting goals that are too ambitious

_____ Bad weather

_____ A lack of motivation

_____ Health problems (identify): _____

_____ Other: _____

_____

Look back at the items you checked. First, identify the problems you've had in the past that no longer apply. Cross them off. (For example, child care may have been a major problem in the past, but now your children are old enough that you can leave them at home unattended.)

Now look for past problems that don't apply to the LEVITY program in particular. For example, walking for 20 minutes at a brisk pace may be less strenuous than previous exercise attempts, so it is a more realistic goal. Cross off these obstacles as well.

If any difficulties still remain, make a specific plan for how you're going to eliminate, work around, or cope with each one. For every problem there is a solution. If you can't think of how to deal with a particular problem, ask family and friends to brainstorm with you. Often, other people can identify options that you have overlooked. Try out some of the options. You may be surprised that the solution is easier than you think.

EXAMPLE:

Unresolved Problem: *I have no one to watch the children while I walk.*

Plan: *I'm going to take my kids to the high school track and place them in the middle with toys to keep them amused as I walk around the track.*

Unresolved Problem: _____

_____

Plan: _____

_____

_____

_____

_____

_____

Unresolved Problem: _____

_____

Plan: _____

_____

_____

_____

_____

_____

Chapter 9

Taking Your LEVITY Vitamins and Minerals

The Nutrients You Need to Relieve the Body Blues

The easiest part of the LEVITY program will be taking your daily supplement. It requires just a few seconds of your time and very little effort. The only work that's involved is deciding what to buy and then developing a simple strategy to make sure you take the tablets regularly.

First, if you are presently taking nutritional supplements, look to see if you're already taking any amount of vitamins B_1 (thiamin), B_2 (riboflavin), or B_6 (pyridoxine); folic acid; vitamin D; or selenium. (If you are taking calcium supplements, check to see if they contain any vitamin D.) The reason for checking is that you want to make sure that adding the LEVITY formula to your current regimen will not put you above the tolerable upper limit, or UL, for any of the ingredients. To help you figure this out, refer to the table "Are You within the Tolerable Upper Limits?" on page 138.

If adding the LEVITY formula to your current intake exceeds the tolerable upper limits, then either stop taking the supplements you are already taking or buy the ingredients in the LEVITY formula individually, leaving out the ones that would put you over the limit.

If you want to buy the LEVITY™ Mood-Elevating Formula (the tablets used in our study), turn to page 160 of the book for ordering information or look for the product at your local health food store, pharmacy, or grocery store.

If you want to purchase the ingredients separately, you will have to buy several products. (We are not aware of any commercial supplement that has all the LEVITY formula ingredients in the recommended amounts in a single tablet, other than the one we had designed specifically for our study.) One solution is to purchase a B-complex tablet that contains 50 milligrams each of

137

Are You within the Tolerable Upper Limits?

To determine whether or not you're below the tolerable upper limits of the six LEVITY ingredients, use this handy table. Write the amounts of the vitamins and minerals you are presently taking in the spaces provided in the second column. Add to this the amount in the LEVITY formula (itemized in the third column). The sum of these two numbers should not exceed the tolerable upper limit, or UL, listed in the final column.

For example, if you are now taking a daily vitamin tablet that contains 2 milligrams of vitamin B_6, adding the 50 milligrams in the LEVITY formula to this amount is only 52 milligrams, which is below the upper limit of 100 milligrams listed in the fourth column.

Ingredients	Amount You Are Currently Taking	Amount in LEVITY Formula	Tolerable Upper Limit
Vitamin B_1 (thiamin)	—— milligrams	50 milligrams	Total amount —— **UL not established. To be conservative, do not exceed 100 milligrams.**
Vitamin B_2 (riboflavin)	—— milligrams	50 milligrams	Total amount —— **UL not established. To be conservative, do not exceed 100 milligrams.**
Vitamin B_6 (pyridoxine)	—— milligrams	50 milligrams	Total amount —— **Do not exceed 100 milligrams.**
Folic acid	—— micrograms	400 micrograms	Total amount —— **Do not exceed 1,000 micrograms.**
Vitamin D	—— IU	400 IU	Total amount —— **Do not exceed 2,000 IU.**
Selenium	—— micrograms	200 micrograms	Total amount —— **Do not exceed 400 micrograms.**

vitamins B_1, B_2, B_6 and 400 micrograms of folic acid. Then all you have to do is purchase the selenium and vitamin D separately. If the B-complex formula does not contain folic acid, then you will need to purchase a folic acid supplement as well.

Remembering to Take Your Vitamins

Most of our 112 volunteers had no difficulty remembering to take their tablets. One of the reasons is that we gave everyone pillboxes with separate compartments for each day of the week. We suggested that they fill the pillbox once a week and place it where it was visible. Most women kept their pillbox in the bathroom or kitchen. A few kept it in a purse or desk drawer at work. One woman who said that she could never remember to take pills balanced her pillbox on top of her toothbrush so she would have to come into contact with it every day. Because the pillboxes worked so well for our volunteers, I recommend that you use one as well. Most pharmacies carry them, and some give them away for free.

Advice for People Who Don't Like to Take Pills

Many of my patients at the University of Washington Women's Health Care Clinic say that they don't like to take pills. To find a solution, I've found that it helps to uncover the precise reason for their aversion. Some women have a hard time swallowing pills, especially large capsules. Some associate all pills with medicine. Some are taking a number of pills to begin with and don't want to add any more. Some fear that taking pills makes them look like a hypochondriac or indicates that they are unwell. Some are worried about possible reactions to the medications, especially stomach upset.

Each problem requires a separate solution. For people who have trouble swallowing pills, I suggest that they first drink a glass of water to lubricate their throats. For some women, this alone removes their difficulties. If necessary, cut the pills in half or grind them with a pill crusher.

When women are worried about the number of pills they are taking, I work with them to see if all their pills are necessary. If they are, then I suggest that they divide them up and take them at different meals.

One of the women I coached in the LEVITY study mentioned that she had a reluctance to take all pills in general. Talking about the problem for just a few minutes helped her see that pills brought to mind images of her mother who had to take a half-dozen pills a day because of a heart condition. As a re-

The Value of a Pillbox

"I USED TO TAKE VITAMINS passively, when I remembered it. Now I'm really conscious about it. The pillbox helps."

LEVITY volunteer, 67

sult, the woman equated pills with illness. When she realized that taking the LEVITY formula was going to improve her mood and perhaps *decrease* her risk of cardiovascular disease, she began to think of them as a road to health, not an indicator of disease.

Possible Side Effects

Only a few women in our study reported any side effects from taking the LEVITY formula, other than the fact that their urine turned a bright orange-yellow color, which is the result of taking 50 milligrams of vitamin B_2. (This is expected and is of no concern.) A few women who took the tablet on an empty stomach experienced a momentary queasiness. (Some in the placebo group mentioned that they felt queasy or dizzy from taking their tablets, even though their tablets contained no active ingredients.) When women experienced mild stomach upset, we advised them to take the tablet along with a meal, which solved the problem for most of them. One woman who felt she was "very sensitive" to B vitamins divided the tablet in half and took it at two separate meals.

When should you take the tablets? Any time of the day is fine unless doing so on an empty stomach makes you feel queasy. In that case, try taking them with a meal. If you take the tablets with the same meal or at the same time every day, you will find they become a part of your daily routine.

Questions and Answers

Q. Will I get any mood benefits from taking the LEVITY formula if I don't go for walks or get added light?

A. We did not test the three components of the LEVITY program individually, so we do not know from our own work if the formula is effective all by itself. But as you learned in chapter 6, other studies have found that each of the individual ingredients can improve mood. Taking all six of them together is likely to have an even greater effect.

Nonetheless, we still recommend that you take part in all three LEVITY program activities. Some of the symptoms of the Body Blues, including overeating and weight gain, appear to respond better to light and exercise than they do to vitamins.

Q. I'm taking a daily multivitamin tablet. Can I continue to take it along with the LEVITY formula?

A. Most one-a-day supplements give you only minimal amounts of the most essential vitamins. Adding the LEVITY formula to such low doses will not exceed tolerable upper limits.

Q. I thought that vitamin B_{12} was also good for your mood. Why didn't you include it in your formula?

A. There are many ingredients in addition to those in the LEVITY formula that may improve your energy level and mood, including vitamin B_{12}, niacin, calcium, iron, docosahexaenoic acid (DHA), and vitamin C. We did not include all of the possible mood-elevating ingredients in our formula because at the time we were planning the study, many of them had not been tested in randomized, double-blind studies. Also, increasing the number of nutrients would have made the formula bulkier and more expensive. But we know of no contraindications of taking other vitamins and minerals with the LEVITY formula as long as you do not exceed the tolerable upper limits.

Q. If I take your LEVITY formula, will I be getting all the vitamins and minerals I need for optimum health?

A. If you are eating a healthy diet and do not have special needs, you will be able to get most of the nutrients you need from food alone. Taking higher amounts of certain vitamins and minerals has been shown to be beneficial for health, but this is a discussion that is beyond the scope of this book.

Q. Why didn't you include St. John's wort or s-adenosylmethionine (SAM-e) in your formula? Aren't they natural substances that have been proven to treat depression in women?

A. When we devised the formula, our goal was to identify nutrients that augmented the body's natural processes. St. John's wort, although a substance found in nature, is not a part of the body's normal biochemical processes. Indeed, it functions very much like a selective serotonin reuptake inhibitor (SSRI) in that it appears to block the uptake of serotonin. You might call it a natural substance with a druglike mechanism.

SAM-e supplements, on the other hand, are supposedly identical to the SAM-e we produce in our own bodies, but the pills can be quite expensive.

To add the amount proven to be effective in clinical trials would have greatly increased the cost of the LEVITY formula. If you want to add these supplements to your regimen, talk with a naturopathic physician, nutritionist, or other specially trained health care provider.

Q. Can I take the vitamins along with antidepressants?

A. You certainly can. In fact, the four B-complex ingredients in the formula have been shown to make antidepressants more effective. As a result, some people may be able to reduce the dose of their medication. (Always consult your health care practitioner before making changes in prescribed medications.)

Q. You mention that the LEVITY formula contains vitamin D$_3$. Does it have to be in that particular form? What is the difference between the various types of vitamin D?

A. Vitamin D$_3$ (cholecalciferol) has the same chemical structure as the nutrient we get from sunlight. Vitamin D$_2$ (ergosterol) comes from plants. For humans, there is no practical difference between vitamins D$_2$ and D$_3$, and the general term *vitamin D* applies to both. We used D$_3$ because it was used in one of the studies that we relied upon to create the formula.

Q. Can I take smaller amounts of the LEVITY nutrients and still see benefits?

A. It is likely that smaller doses will have some effect on your mood, especially if you are deficient in them. But we can only vouch for the amounts used in our study.

Your Turn

If you have had difficulty remembering to take supplements in the past, complete the exercises that follow. They will help you identify why you've experienced problems before and will help you figure out the best ways to overcome them.

Exercise 1. Identify Your Barriers to Taking the LEVITY Supplements

Following are some of the most common reasons for not taking supplements. Check the ones that apply to you. (There is space at the bottom to add additional items.)

I've had the following problems taking supplements:

_____ Not knowing whether I've taken them
_____ Not knowing where they are
_____ Forgetting to take them altogether
_____ Forgetting to take them on trips
_____ Having unusually strong reactions to taking pills
_____ Not knowing if they're really necessary
_____ Running out of them and neglecting to get more
_____ I don't like taking pills in general
_____ Other: _____

_____

_____

Exercise 2. Overcoming Obstacles

Look over the list above. If you checked any of the items, make a plan for solving each problem in the area provided below.

EXAMPLE:

Problem: *I don't like the thought of taking pills because I don't like to swallow them.*

Plan: *I will cut the tablet in half and take it with yogurt. If that doesn't work, I'll get a pill crusher and mix the pill with the yogurt.*

Problem #1: _____

_____

Plan: _____

_____

_____

Problem #2: _____

_____

Plan: _____

_____

_____

Problem #3: _____

_____

Plan: _____

_____

_____

Chapter 10

LEVITY for Life

*Making Light, Exercise, and Essential Nutrients
a Central Part of Your Life*

As you have learned, each of the components of the LEVITY program—light, exercise, and the six essential vitamins and minerals—has been proven in independent studies to relieve some aspect of the Body Blues. For example, light increases your energy, brightens your mood, clears your mind, relieves sleep problems, and reduces your appetite. Moderate-intensity exercise gives you all of these benefits plus it lowers your anxiety, tones your muscles, burns excess fat and calories, buffers the effects of stress, and gives you a sense of pride and accomplishment. The LEVITY formula gives you the raw ingredients you need to make the mood-enhancing chemicals triggered by bright light and exercise.

When all three components are combined into one program, they address all 10 of the most common symptoms of the Body Blues.

- Eating too much and gaining weight
- Low energy
- Difficulty concentrating
- Sleep difficulties
- Irritability or tension
- Daytime drowsiness
- Decreased interest in sex
- Mild anxiety
- Mild depression
- Heightened sensitivity to rejection or criticism

There is another benefit to combining the three elements into one program: One of the activities may help compensate for the possible negative effects of another. For example, as discussed in chapter 7, spending more time in the sun boosts your mood and tames your appetite, but it also increases your exposure to ultraviolet (UV) light. Blocking the light with protective clothing or sunscreen is not an ideal solution because it deprives you of the mood-enhancing effects of vitamin D, which is created whenever sun shines on your bare skin. The way out of this dilemma is to block the sun as you normally would but get your vitamin D in supplement form. The LEVITY formula supplies this important vitamin. In addition, three of its other ingredients—selenium, vitamin B_2, and folic acid—have been shown to offer protection against UV light.[1] Thus, the risk of getting more sunlight is reduced by taking the LEVITY supplement.

Similarly, the supplement also prevents possible vitamin deficiencies that can result from becoming more physically active. Exercise increases the need for vitamins B_1, B_2, and B_6, nutrients required to provide energy and build muscle. B-vitamin deficiency is more likely in people who eat fewer than 2,000 calories a day, which includes a majority of women. But you won't have to worry that going for frequent walks or cutting back on calories will rob you of these important vitamins, because they are included in your daily supplement.

As you can see, the three activities in the LEVITY program have a synergistic effect. Together, they address more symptoms of the Body Blues than any one alone, and they also compensate for each other's possible negative effects. Yet, the three activities combined do not take any extra time or effort than one of them alone. For example, it doesn't take you any more time to walk outdoors than to walk on an indoor treadmill, yet exercising outdoors gives you the combined benefits of light *and* exercise. Taking the LEVITY supplement requires only a few extra seconds each day. In essence, the LEVITY program relies on "multitasking" to save you time and energy.

The LEVITY Program—A Better Way to Live

When you've been on the LEVITY program for 6 to 8 weeks, you will have made great strides in relieving your Body Blues. You'll feel lighter in mood, lighter on your feet, less stressed, and more positive about the future. Because you will have found a reliable way to produce mood-enhancing chemicals, you will be less likely to turn to food for comfort. You will also have a greater sense of empowerment because you will be relieving your symptoms through your own effort and determination.

As time goes on, you may begin to see that the LEVITY program is more than an 8-week solution to the Body Blues—it's a healthier way to live. One of our volunteers sent us this e-mail message about a year after the study had ended:

> *I think the program has given me some structure, some strength to just go ahead and do what I've known was good for me all along. I've always known that light and exercise made me feel better, but I needed the program to make me do it. Now, the walks, the outdoor activity, and the vitamins are a part of my ongoing life. It's a good feeling to be doing what I know is best.*

How can *you* turn the LEVITY program into a permanent lifestyle change? Some of this will happen automatically. For example, after you've been on the program for a few months, you won't have to remind yourself to get out and walk because it will have become an ingrained habit. In fact, you may feel "twitchy" if you haven't been able to exercise. Staying inside all day on a sunny day will seem as foreign to you as living in a cave. Taking your daily LEVITY supplement will also have become a matter of routine.

To reinforce these behaviors even more, factor them in when you make long-term plans. For example, you may now live in an area where you have to drive 10 miles to get to a safe and pleasant place to walk. The next time you move, look for a house or apartment near a park, walking trail, lake, or gym so that you can open the door and start walking. If your present home is dark inside, make sure that the next house or apartment is flooded with natural light. If your current friends are not interested in going for walks, cultivate new ones who are. When it's time to replace a lightbulb, invest in a brighter and more energy efficient subcompact fluorescent bulb. The more you build your life around light and exercise, the more energetic, healthy, trim, and high-spirited you will be.

Anticipating and Managing Setbacks

No matter how dedicated you are to getting more light and exercise, there will be times in the months and years to come when you will fall back into your old habits. You can count on it. It's human nature to return to old ways, especially during times of stress or transition.

Of the three activities in the LEVITY program, the one you are likely to find most difficult to sustain is getting regular exercise. Exercise takes time and effort. Furthermore, once we reach adulthood, it's not programmed into our genes. Until the last 100 or so years, people lived physically demanding lives. Bringing in food, preserving it for the winter, finding fuel, building shelters, making and caring for clothes, taking care of children, and traveling from place to place forced people to be physically active most of the time. When the day's work was done, they didn't have the time, energy, or *need* to go for a 20-minute brisk walk. They just wanted to relax. Those adults who had an inborn need to keep exercising once the work was done would not have survived. "Take care of your survival needs and then rest" seems to be a prime directive.

To survive in the industrialized world, however, requires very little physical energy. We no longer have to devote an entire day of the week to the laundry; we can dispense with the chore during a few commercial breaks on TV. We don't have to make six loaves of bread each week; we can simply pick up the bread at the store. Many jobs demand that we sit in one location for hours on end, exercising only our vocal cords and fingers. We can surmount the highest hills and crisscross the entire nation just by hanging on to a steering wheel and depressing the accelerator of a car. And yet, we are still programmed to rest whenever possible. For the first time in human history, we have to find *artificial* ways to get enough exercise simply to maintain our mental and physical health.

The LEVITY program helps give you the structure and motivation you need to become more active. But there will be times when you lapse back into a more sedentary mode. Some days, you will be so pressured that you cannot carve even 20 minutes from your schedule. Or the weather might be so miserable that you have to stay indoors for days or weeks at a time. Or an accident, illness, or other misfortune may keep you from walking. Simply going through the fall and winter holiday season can be enough to derail you. For weeks, you are busier than ever and surrounded by rich, delectable food. You do too much, eat too much, and skimp on your walks. Then comes January and the holiday excitement is over. You may feel like hibernating until spring.

There is an entire field of study called relapse prevention, which is devoted to helping people cope with setbacks such as these. One of the insights to come out of this research is that it's not just stress, busyness, and adversity that make people abandon their healthy habits. It's also the feeling that they've lost control. Something has happened to them that they didn't predict or were not able to avoid. They've lost the sense that they can make a difference in their own lives. When people feel powerless about improving their state of being, they tend to fall back into dysfunctional behaviors, especially those that deliver instant gratification. Although going for a brisk walk can improve your mood in just 10 minutes, your favorite chocolate dessert can make you feel better just by *thinking* about it.

Starting Over

When you reach a low point, there's only one thing to do: cut your losses and start over. Mastering the art of starting over is one of life's most valuable skills. The celebrated inventor Thomas Edison created more than 800 different lightbulb filaments that failed before he created one that worked. On average, smokers have to quit smoking three times before breaking the habit for good. Those who quit trying after the first or second failed attempt never reach their goal. It's people with the determination and humility to start over and over and over and *over* who finally succeed.

So it is with the LEVITY program. *The key to making exercise and light a central part of your life is to start over again each and every time that you lapse.* The Japanese word *shoshin* means "beginner's mind." This is the state of mind that allows you to see the world afresh, for the first time every time. When you begin the LEVITY program for the fourth time in as many years, think of it as a brand-new adventure. Experience the joy of restoring your energy and peace of mind all over again, just as you did the very first time.

All-or-Nothing Thinking

The opposite of having a beginner's mind is to be trapped in all-or-nothing thinking or to be so intent on attaining perfection that you give up at the first hint of failure. One of the women I coached in the LEVITY study injured her knee in a fall down a flight of stairs. She had to stop walking for several weeks to allow it to heal. Since she couldn't walk, she told herself, there was no point in doing the other two parts of the program. She had blown it.

With my encouragement, she decided to go back to taking her supplements and getting more light. As soon as she was given the go-ahead by her physical therapist, she began taking slow walks around the block. When the program was over, I was pleased to see that her mood had improved significantly over the course of the study. By abandoning her all-or-nothing thinking, she had been able to benefit from the program.

A Broad and Forgiving Path

When I think about all that's involved in creating and maintaining healthy habits, I envision a broad path with a white stripe down the middle and ditches on either side. Many people think that they have to tread the white line or they've failed. But it's not possible to walk such a narrow line without wavering. Most people toe the line some of the time, wander off to the edges some of the time, and fall into the ditch some of the time. Although some of these places feel decidedly better than others, they are all part of the same broad and forgiving path.

In the future, when you find that *you've* strayed from the centerline, dispense with the guilt, shame, and self-incrimination. They get you nowhere. And don't think about all the times that you've failed in the past. Instead, count the number of times you've gathered the strength to start over. Then plot a new course that takes you back to the center. You are on the LEVITY program *as long as you keep returning to the three activities each and every time that you lapse.*

Admittedly, the hardest time to start over again is when you've been mired in the ditch for a period of time. You've stopped exercising. You're snacking at night once again. You've run out of your supplements and haven't replaced them. Maybe you've gained back all the weight that you've lost. At these times, you may need outside support.

To rebuild your momentum, consider rereading parts of this book. In particular, I recommend that you review your answers to the first exercise in chapter 8, "What Are Your Reasons for Exercising?" (see page 132). If you bring to mind all the rewards that you get from moderate-intensity exercise, you may rekindle your interest in starting over again. I also recommend that you seek the support of your health care provider. (Many health insurance programs now pay for what are called health promotion visits.) I am always gratified when a patient makes an appointment just to get support and suggestions for creating a healthier life.

Your friends can be very helpful as well. For example, for years I'd been intending to take a yoga class, but I never got around to it. During a walk with a friend, I talked about my lack of follow-through. Although she herself did not practice yoga, she explained why she thought it would be especially valuable for me. Her insight and encouragement were enough to put me over the edge and sign up for a class.

If you continue to have problems with sustaining your motivation, take a long, hard look at your life. What is it that keeps pulling you away from the centerline? Maybe your relationship with your partner or parent is causing you stress. Maybe you have drifted away from the activities that nourish your soul. Maybe you are weighed down by loneliness and haven't gone to enough effort to create new friends. To get a clearer sense of what is holding you back, consider working with a supportive therapist or participating in personal growth activities.

Once you've lightened your load, begin the three activities in the LEVITY program as if it were the very first time. Reward yourself for beginning anew. To make a relapse less likely, have someone take pictures of you while you are exercising and post the pictures where you will see them. Think of yourself as an active person. When circumstances intervene and you can't walk for several days in a row, tell yourself, "I am an active person who happens to be not exercising for these few days." Every aspect of your being will benefit from your persistence.

A Look to the Future

In the months and years to come, scientists will keep expanding our knowledge of the intricate connections between gender and mood. In particular, the links between hormones, brain chemicals, and receptors will become ever clearer. In addition, the influence that light, exercise, and essential nutrients have on those systems will become better known. Meanwhile, pharmaceutical companies will be using all those new discoveries to devise more effective medications with fewer side effects. The drugs that will be available 20 years from now will seem miraculous compared with the ones we have today.

But even when highly effective medications for the Body Blues become available, there will still be many women who prefer to solve their fatigue, stress, and eating problems by creating a healthier lifestyle. The most effective changes today and in the future are likely to be those that help restore a more natural environment and set of behaviors. Getting enough bright light, exercise, and essential nutrients will be as important in 2050 as they are today.

I wish you well!

PART 4

Resources
and
References

Your LEVITY Journal

In the pages that follow, you will find a simple journal to help you keep track of the three activities of the LEVITY program. Each day of the week you can record (1) the amount of time you are exposed to outdoor light (or bright indoor light), (2) the number of minutes that you exercised, and (3) the fact that you have taken your daily LEVITY supplements.

There is also a space to record daily comments. You can write down whatever you wish in this section, including changes of mood, stressful or uplifting events, or changes in your health. I recommend that you also write down all the successes you are having with the program. For example, if you have exercised 5 days a week for an entire month, take a moment to record that fact. When you notice a difference in the intensity or frequency of a particular symptom such as overeating, consider recording that accomplishment as well.

There will be some days when you do not meet all your goals. This is to be expected. Instead of blaming yourself or feeling that you've failed, use your problem-solving skills to surmount your obstacles. On each day of the journal, there is a space to record what you plan to do differently tomorrow. For example, if you didn't have time to exercise one day, describe what you plan to do the next day to squeeze it in. Be specific. Instead of making a vague statement such as "I will find time to exercise," write down what you plan to do: "I will set my alarm clock 20 minutes earlier so I can walk before going to work."

At the bottom of the comment section is a list of the days of the menstrual cycle. If you are having menstrual periods, circling the appropriate day will help you see whether your moods are linked with any particular part of the cycle. (Consider Day 1 as the day that bleeding begins.)

You have our permission to photocopy a blank page of the LEVITY journal so you can keep an ongoing record in the months to come. (You can also visit www.thebodyblues.com and download a blank journal page from the Web.) Or you can create your own journal, customizing the pages in numerous ways, such as adding more space for comments, including a place to record other information like your weight or how many calories you've consumed, or adding inspirational messages.

Some people do not like to keep journals. (A small percentage of women in the LEVITY study found journal keeping a chore rather than a helpful tool.) If you do not want to keep a journal, I urge you to find some way to record your completion of the program assignments. Just jot a quick note in your day planner, personal digital assistant, or calendar. You can simply write down the initial *L* when you've been exposed to bright outdoor or indoor light, *E* when you've exercised 20 minutes or more, and *V* when you've taken your supplement. Research shows that when you are beginning to practice new and healthier habits, recording your activities makes it more likely that you will follow through with the program.

Day of the week: _____   **Date:** _____

Light   _____ Minutes spent outdoors (or exposed to very bright indoor light)

Exercise   _____ Minutes of brisk outdoor walking (or other moderately intense exercise)

Vitamins   ❏   LEVITY formula

Comments and successes: _____

_____

_____

What, if anything, do I want to do differently tomorrow? _____

_____

_____

Circle day of menstrual cycle (if applicable):
1 2 3 4 5 6 7 8 9 10 11 12 13 14 15 16 17 18
19 20 21 22 23 24 25 26 27 28 29 30 31

Day of the week: _____ **Date:** _____

Light _____ Minutes spent outdoors (or exposed to very bright indoor light)

Exercise _____ Minutes of brisk outdoor walking (or other moderately intense exercise)

Vitamins ☐ LEVITY formula

Comments and successes: _____
_____
_____
_____

What, if anything, do I want to do differently tomorrow? _____
_____
_____

Circle day of menstrual cycle (if applicable):
1   2   3   4   5   6   7   8   9   10   11   12   13   14   15   16   17   18
19   20   21   22   23   24   25   26   27   28   29   30   31

Day of the week: _____ **Date:** _____

Light _____ Minutes spent outdoors (or exposed to very bright indoor light)

Exercise _____ Minutes of brisk outdoor walking (or other moderately intense exercise)

Vitamins ☐ LEVITY formula

Comments and successes: _____
_____
_____
_____

What, if anything, do I want to do differently tomorrow? _____
_____
_____

Circle day of menstrual cycle (if applicable):
1   2   3   4   5   6   7   8   9   10   11   12   13   14   15   16   17   18
19   20   21   22   23   24   25   26   27   28   29   30   31

Day of the week: _____   **Date:** _____

Light   _____ Minutes spent outdoors (or exposed to very bright indoor light)

Exercise   _____ Minutes of brisk outdoor walking (or other moderately intense exercise)

Vitamins   ☐   LEVITY formula

Comments and successes: _____
_____
_____
_____

What, if anything, do I want to do differently tomorrow? _____
_____
_____

Circle day of menstrual cycle (if applicable):
1   2   3   4   5   6   7   8   9   10   11   12   13   14   15   16   17   18
19   20   21   22   23   24   25   26   27   28   29   30   31

Day of the week: _____   **Date:** _____

Light   _____ Minutes spent outdoors (or exposed to very bright indoor light)

Exercise   _____ Minutes of brisk outdoor walking (or other moderately intense exercise)

Vitamins   ☐   LEVITY formula

Comments and successes: _____
_____
_____
_____

What, if anything, do I want to do differently tomorrow? _____
_____
_____

Circle day of menstrual cycle (if applicable):
1   2   3   4   5   6   7   8   9   10   11   12   13   14   15   16   17   18
19   20   21   22   23   24   25   26   27   28   29   30   31

Day of the week: _____   **Date:** _____

Light   _____ Minutes spent outdoors (or exposed to very bright indoor light)

Exercise   _____ Minutes of brisk outdoor walking (or other moderately intense exercise)

Vitamins   ☐   LEVITY formula

Comments and successes: _____
_____
_____
_____

What, if anything, do I want to do differently tomorrow? _____
_____
_____

Circle day of menstrual cycle (if applicable):
1 2 3 4 5 6 7 8 9 10 11 12 13 14 15 16 17 18
19 20 21 22 23 24 25 26 27 28 29 30 31

Day of the week: _____   **Date:** _____

Light   _____ Minutes spent outdoors (or exposed to very bright indoor light)

Exercise   _____ Minutes of brisk outdoor walking (or other moderately intense exercise)

Vitamins   ☐   LEVITY formula

Comments and successes: _____
_____
_____
_____

What, if anything, do I want to do differently tomorrow? _____
_____
_____

Circle day of menstrual cycle (if applicable):
1 2 3 4 5 6 7 8 9 10 11 12 13 14 15 16 17 18
19 20 21 22 23 24 25 26 27 28 29 30 31

Day of the week: _____   **Date:** _____

Light   _____ Minutes spent outdoors (or exposed to very bright indoor light)

Exercise   _____ Minutes of brisk outdoor walking (or other moderately intense exercise)

Vitamins   ☐   LEVITY formula

Comments and successes: _____
_____
_____
_____

What, if anything, do I want to do differently tomorrow? _____
_____
_____

Circle day of menstrual cycle (if applicable):
1   2   3   4   5   6   7   8   9   10   11   12   13   14   15   16   17   18
19   20   21   22   23   24   25   26   27   28   29   30   31

Day of the week: _____   **Date:** _____

Light   _____ Minutes spent outdoors (or exposed to very bright indoor light)

Exercise   _____ Minutes of brisk outdoor walking (or other moderately intense exercise)

Vitamins   ☐   LEVITY formula

Comments and successes: _____
_____
_____
_____

What, if anything, do I want to do differently tomorrow? _____
_____
_____

Circle day of menstrual cycle (if applicable):
1   2   3   4   5   6   7   8   9   10   11   12   13   14   15   16   17   18
19   20   21   22   23   24   25   26   27   28   29   30   31

Day of the week: _____   **Date:** _____

Light   _____ Minutes spent outdoors (or exposed to very bright indoor light)

Exercise   _____ Minutes of brisk outdoor walking (or other moderately intense exercise)

Vitamins   ❐   LEVITY formula

Comments and successes: _____
_____
_____
_____

What, if anything, do I want to do differently tomorrow? _____
_____
_____

Circle day of menstrual cycle (if applicable):
1 2 3 4 5 6 7 8 9 10 11 12 13 14 15 16 17 18
19 20 21 22 23 24 25 26 27 28 29 30 31

Day of the week: _____   **Date:** _____

Light   _____ Minutes spent outdoors (or exposed to very bright indoor light)

Exercise   _____ Minutes of brisk outdoor walking (or other moderately intense exercise)

Vitamins   ❐   LEVITY formula

Comments and successes: _____
_____
_____
_____

What, if anything, do I want to do differently tomorrow? _____
_____
_____

Circle day of menstrual cycle (if applicable):
1 2 3 4 5 6 7 8 9 10 11 12 13 14 15 16 17 18
19 20 21 22 23 24 25 26 27 28 29 30 31

Where to Find Vitamins, Lighting Products, and Exercise Gear

The LEVITY program requires no equipment or supplies, apart from the daily supplement and a good pair of walking shoes. But there are a few products that may make the program more enjoyable for you or help you adapt it to your needs. For example, you might want to expand your lighting options by purchasing a light box. Or you might want your own lux meter so you can locate areas in your home or workplace that need more light. Or you might enjoy exercising to special walking tapes designed to entertain you *and* keep you within your target heart range.

You will find information about these products and more in this resource section. For specific, up-to-the-minute recommendations and Web links, visit www.thebodyblues.com. (If you are not connected to the Internet, you can use a computer at your local library. Most libraries have special programs to help you learn Internet basics.)

If you find additional products that help you enjoy and stick with the LEVITY program, please let me know so I can share them with others. Send me an e-mail at: drbrown@thebodyblues.com.

Vitamins and Minerals

The LEVITY formula. The supplements that we created for the LEVITY study are now commercially available in a single, easy-to-swallow tablet. Ask for the LEVITY™ Mood-Elevating Formula at your local health food store, pharmacy, or supermarket. The LEVITY formula can also be purchased directly from Geneva Health and Nutrition, a manufacturer of supplements for women's health. Orders can be placed online at www.geneva-health.com or via their toll-free ordering line, (800) 947-8482. Geneva can also be contacted via e-mail at info@geneva-health.com.

The LEVITY Journal

Many of the volunteers in the LEVITY study enjoyed the support and encouragement they got from jotting down their program activities in a daily journal. You can purchase the LEVITY Journal in an attractive 3-ring translucent binder. The journal includes inspirational quotations, supportive comments from LEVITY participants, and a daily symptom diary (as described on page 153). The price is $20. (Refills are available.)

To order online, visit www.thestoreforhealthyliving.com, or send a check for $26 (includes USPS Priority Mailing) to:

The Store for Healthy Living
2401 North Cedar Street
Tacoma, WA 98406

Phototherapy Devices

Light boxes. When you are unable to exercise outdoors during daylight hours or if you want to illuminate a dark office, you may want a solar substitute. Of the numerous light therapy products on the market, light boxes are the most popular. Light boxes are rectangular light fixtures clad in metal or wood that sit on a table or desk. (Common dimensions are 24 × 15 × 4 inches.) The light is supplied by high-intensity fluorescent tubes. Look for a light fixture that is designed to treat winter depression and provides 5,000 to 10,000 lux. Make sure that it is also:

- UL-approved
- UV-shielded
- Flicker-free

Note: Do *not* buy a tanning lamp or a phototherapy device designed to treat psoriasis, because they emit ultraviolet light.

If you want to use a light box while you exercise indoors, consider purchasing a freestanding light box. They are tall enough to shine at head height yet are light and easy to move. (Typically, they cost more than a tabletop model.)

If you want to bring bright light into your workplace, phototherapy desk lamps are ideal. They look like ordinary desk lamps but supply as much as 10,000 lux of light. You can aim the light down at your desk to illuminate your work surface or turn it toward your face to enjoy an in-office light therapy session. Some people appreciate light therapy desk lamps because they don't look like therapeutic devices.

Make sure that you are buying a bright enough lamp, however. Some desk lamps are equipped with full-spectrum bulbs and are advertised to help treat the winter blues, but they emit too little light to affect your mood. Look for products that provide from 5,000 to 10,000 lux of light. (The lux rating will be featured prominently in the advertising.)

If you travel frequently and want to bring along your own light source, look for portable light boxes designed for frequent travelers. If you use these devices at specific times of the day, they can also help you overcome jet lag. (Detailed instructions for preventing jet lag come along with the products.)

For the greatest freedom of movement, look for lighting devices that deliver the advertised amount of light at a distance of 2 feet or more. Some have a therapeutic range of only 12 inches, requiring you to stay very close. If you are 2 feet away from some 10,000-lux light boxes, for example, you may be getting only 2,500 lux of light. If the full 10,000 lux enters your eyes, your therapy session can be as brief as 30 minutes. If the light has been reduced to 2,500 lux by the time it gets to you, it may require a 3-hour session to get the same results.

Lights with a shorter therapeutic range can be effective, although you must leave them on for several hours. This may not be a problem if you work at a desk for much of your workday. (As I remarked earlier, it is possible to get so much bright artificial light that you feel tense or jittery or even experience a low-level mania. Don't overdo it.)

All lighting devices should come with a money-back guarantee. The lightbulbs are long-lasting but should be replaced every 2 to 3 years, because they diminish greatly in intensity over time.

Light visors. Another option is a light visor. This is baseball-type cap equipped with tiny UV-shielded lights that shine into your eyes. The light is not as bright as a light box, but it is so close to your field of vision that it has been shown to be equally effective. Light visors allow you to wander freely about your house and can be taken on trips as a treatment for jet lag or simply as a portable light source.

Dawn simulators. A third type of phototherapy device to consider is a dawn simulator. These lamps sit beside your bed and wake you up with a glow of light that gradually increases in intensity. They operate on the theory that light that mimics the natural onset of dawn can reset the body's circadian rhythm and relieve vegetative symptoms. Several studies suggest that they are effective for treating seasonal affective disorder (SAD). You can either purchase a lamp with electronic controls or plug an ordinary (nonfluorescent) lamp into a special electrical box that controls the intensity and timing of the light. Brand names include SunRizr, SunUp, the SunRise Alarm Clock, and the Rise and Shine Alarm Clock.

Some health insurance companies reimburse their clients for the purchase of light boxes if they are deemed necessary to treat medical conditions such as SAD, sleep problems, PMS, and problems adapting to shift work. Your health care provider will need to fill out a form specifying the appropriate diagnostic code and reason for prescribing the device.

To purchase lighting devices, you have many resources. In many metropolitan areas, especially those in the northern tier of states, specialty lighting stores carry light therapy products. Seattle and other northern cities have stores devoted exclusively to these devices. (Look in the yellow pages of your phone book under the heading "Lightbulbs" or "Lighting fixtures.") If you can't find what you are looking for in your local area, turn to the Internet. Search for phrases such as "light therapy products," "winter blues," "seasonal affective disorder," and "light boxes." You can also visit www.thebodyblues.com for specific recommendations.

The following company has a full range of phototherapy devices:

Light Therapy Products
6125 Ives Lane North
Plymouth, MN 55442
(800) 486-6723
www.lighttherapyproducts.com

Cost-Effective, Energy-Efficient Indoor Lighting

One of the keys to relieving the Body Blues is to bring more natural daylight into your home. One option is to install sun tubes. Also called light tubes or sun pipes, these highly reflective pipes run from your roof down to a ceiling fixture with a diffuser that broadens the area of illumination. Sun tubes offer a number of advantages over other sources of daylight.

- They provide glare-free light that doesn't contribute to summer heat buildup.
- The light is UV-shielded so fabrics will not fade.
- They can be installed in areas of your home where ordinary windows or skylights would be impractical.

Sun tubes range from 8 to 40 inches in diameter. The bigger the diameter, the greater the area of illumination. The best ones have a UV-protected, polycarbonate dome that projects a few inches above the roof and a highly polished reflective inner coating that reflects 95 percent or more of the light. Suppliers claim that they are as easy to install as a stovepipe and will not leak. (Some suppliers will not provide a warranty against leaks, however, unless they install them.) Inquire at your local hardware or lighting store or search the yellow pages or the Internet for "sun tubes," "light tubes," or "sun pipes." The following supplier has sun tubes and a wide range of other indoor lighting products:

Indoor Lighting at a Glance

This chart summarizes the benefits and drawbacks of all four types of indoor lighting. Refer to the information below when selecting the most cost-effective, energy-efficient products to brighten your indoor environment.

Type of Light	Efficiency	Life Span (in hours)
Incandescent (ordinary lightbulbs)	Waste 90 percent of energy consumed	750 to 1,000
Halogen	25 percent more efficient than incandescent lighting	1,000 to 2,000
Fluorescent tubes	400 percent more efficient than incandescent lighting	11,000 to 18,000
Subcompact fluorescents	400 percent more efficient than incandescent lighting	10,000 to 18,000

Jade Mountain, Inc.
PO Box 4616
Boulder, CO 80306-4616
(800) 442-1972
www.jademountain.com

In addition to bringing more natural light into your home, you may wish to add more artificial light as well. There are four basic sources of indoor artificial lighting.

- Incandescent bulbs
- Halogen bulbs
- Fluorescent tubes
- Subcompact fluorescent bulbs

Incandescent bulbs are the familiar lightbulbs that have changed very little since they were invented by Thomas Edison in 1879. Incandescent bulbs

Benefits/Comments	Drawbacks
Bulbs give a full range of wattage and fit ordinary fixtures. Best for closets and other places where lights are turned on briefly.	They have a short life span, are inefficient, and contribute to summer heat buildup.
Small size and intense light make these ideal for spot or task lighting.	Bulbs burn so hot that they are a fire hazard; they also emit more ultraviolet light than other light sources.
These are good for illuminating large areas. Available in cool, white, warm, and full-spectrum.	Tubes require special fixtures.
Bulbs are best used in locations where lights are left on for several hours or in hard-to-reach places. Many can be used in ordinary fixtures.	Bulbs are expensive to purchase but save money in the long run. Very bright light is not available at this time (maximum is equivalent to a 150-watt incandescent bulb).

are inexpensive to purchase, but they are not energy efficient. As much as 90 percent of the energy they consume is given off as waste heat.

Halogen lights—those very bright, tiny lights used in some car head-lights, indoor lamps, and torchieres—were once regarded as the lighting of the future because they require less energy and last longer than incandescent bulbs. But they have their limitations as well. They are better for spot and task lighting than general illumination. Also, they burn so hot that they can be a fire hazard.

Fluorescent tube lighting is far more efficient than halogen lights. The new models with improved electronic ballasts do not have the hum, flicker, and un-flattering light characteristic of early fluorescent lights. In addition to linear fluorescent tubes, there are now subcompact fluorescent bulbs. A decade ago, fluorescent bulbs were very expensive ($30 each) and were too big to fit into ordinary light fixtures. Now the prices have fallen and the technology has im-proved to the point that they can be used throughout your home.

For the purposes of the LEVITY program, fluorescent lights are ideal whether you use the familiar linear tubes or subcompact bulbs. They are so energy efficient that you can afford to live in a bright indoor environment.

When you purchase subcompact fluorescent lights for the first time, you will need to adapt your thinking about wattage. For example, you know that a 150-watt incandescent lightbulb is very bright. But a subcompact fluores-cent bulb that gives the same intensity of light draws only 50 watts. The fol-lowing chart will help you make these conversions.

Wattage Conversion

Subcompact Fluorescents		Ordinary Bulbs
14 watts	=	40 watts
20 watts	=	60 watts
25 watts	=	75 watts
32 watts	=	100 watts
50 watts	=	150 watts

For even more savings, look for subcompact fluorescent bulbs that dis-play the Energy Star label. Products with this designation meet strict gov-ernment and industry standards for efficiency and energy conservation. According to government studies, if all Americans used appliances, light-bulbs, and fixtures with the Energy Star label, our national annual energy bill would be reduced by about $200 billion. Go to www.energystar.gov for more information or to locate suppliers in your local area. The site will also alert you to any special sales. (Some utilities offer discount coupons to reward you for purchasing more energy-efficient bulbs.)

Lux meters. These are devices designed to measure the amount of visible light in the environment. A lux meter can help you identify which areas of your home or office are most in need of a "light makeover." It will also help you monitor your progress as you begin to make changes.

Look for a meter that measures light in lux (rather than foot-candles) and has a range from 10 lux or lower to 50,000 lux. You will find them at well-stocked camera stores or by searching the Internet (search for "lux meter"). The prices range from about $60 to several hundred dollars. If you order one of the inexpensive models, make sure that it comes with a money-back guarantee and measures light levels as low as 10 lux. Visit www.thebodyblues.com for specific recommendations.

Resources for Walkers

Heart rate monitors. For some people, a heart rate monitor is a necessity because they find it difficult to take their pulse as they walk. Others like them simply because they eliminate the need to stop and check their pulse—they can just glance down at the digital display. And some people (like me) find that having a monitor makes them more motivated to stay within a particular range.

If you're interested in buying a heart rate monitor, you have a bewildering range of options. All you really need is a simple device that measures your pulse and displays it on a watch. For less than $20, you can purchase one that fits over a finger and uses an optical sensor to detect your heartbeat.

If you wish, you can purchase monitors that have a variety of "bells and whistles." For example, some monitors have preprogrammed exercise sessions. Some models beep or even "talk" to you when you stray outside your target heart range. Other models record all your workout sessions so you can download them onto your computer. Yet others keep track of the miles you've walked and the calories you've burned. And as an added safety feature, some monitors include a panic alarm.

A product especially well-suited for the LEVITY program is the HEARTalker Personal Trainer by Newlife Technologies. This monitor straps around your chest and has a 20-minute preset walking program designed to keep you within 50 to 70 percent of your maximum heart rate, which is the LEVITY walking prescription. A voice "speaks" to you through a set of headphones, telling you if you need to speed up or slow down. It is reasonably priced.

New Life Technologies
One Park West Circle, Suite 303
Midlothian, VA 23113
(800) 915-5566
www.HEARTalker.com

For other heart rate monitors, visit your local athletic or sporting goods store or search the Internet for "heart rate monitors" or "pulse meters."

Walking tapes. Just listening to music can boost your mood. When you combine your favorite music with outdoor walking, you can feel exhilarated. All you need is a portable radio, an audiocassette player, or a CD player. For safety's sake, turn down the volume so you can hear traffic noises and stay aware of your surroundings.

If you'd rather have a more structured music selection, there are special walking tapes, featuring music that has been carefully selected to keep you within your target heart range. You can pick both the type of music and the pace. For example, you can choose from rock, jazz, classical, Christian, show tunes, country, or Big Band music in a variety of target heart ranges.

Typically, the tapes come in three levels of exertion—beginner, intermediate, and advanced. The beginner series may be right for older women, women who have been very sedentary, or those who are significantly overweight. Intermediate tapes are best for the majority of women. Advanced tapes are for younger women or fit women of all ages.

Some walking tapes specify a range of beats per minute. These numbers refer to *musical* beats per minute, not heartbeats per minute. A walking tape with 105 to 110 musical beats per minute, for example, might get your heart up to only 90 beats per minute. You will have to experiment to find the correct pace for you.

To locate walking tapes, go to an athletic store, healthy living store, or search the Internet for "walking tapes," "audio fitness tapes," or "exercise music." The following company has a particularly large collection of walking tapes. (When you reach their home page, search for "walking tapes" on their search engine.)

Collage Video
5390 Main Street NE
Minneapolis, MN 55421
(800) 433-6769
www.collagevideo.com

Audiobooks. If you want your 20-minute walking sessions to fly by, listen to books on audiotape in your favorite genre. As the plot thickens, your walks might lengthen. You can buy the tapes from a bookstore and swap them with friends, rent them from the library, or rent them from an audiotape rental store. You can also download books from the Internet and listen to them on a digital player. Search the Internet for "audiobooks."

High-domed, transparent umbrellas. When it's raining or snowing outside, a transparent umbrella will keep you dry but still let in all the daylight. If the umbrella also has a high dome, you can carry it low over your head for even greater protection, yet still be able to look straight ahead and see where you are going. (As you know, looking straight ahead increases the amount of light that enters your eyes.)

To purchase online, visit www.thestoreforhealthyliving.com. Or mail a check for $29 (includes shipping and handling) to:

The Store for Healthy Living
2401 North Cedar Street
Tacoma, WA 98406

Walking and Outdoor Apparel

Your best chances of finding comfortable walking shoes and sportswear that wicks away moisture are at sporting goods stores or stores that specialize in outdoor wear and recreational equipment. There are even sports apparel stores and Internet sites designed specifically for women. Look in your local yellow pages under "Sporting Goods—Retail" and "Sportswear." Search the Internet for phrases such as "women sportswear," "walking clothes," "sports bras," and "walking gear."

Two popular Internet sites are www.womens-sports.com (888-977-2255) and www.title9sports.com (800-342-4448).

Recommended Reading

- *Changing for Good* by James O. Prochaska, Ph.D. Avon Books, 1995. Dr. Prochaska and two colleagues interviewed more than 1,000 people who were able to change positively and permanently without psychotherapy. They discovered that change does not depend on luck or willpower but on a process that can be learned. This book will provide support and advice for women who have difficulty starting or maintaining the LEVITY program.

• *The Complete Guide to Walking for Health, Weight Loss, and Fitness* by Mark Fenton. Lyons Press, 2001. This book is written for beginning walkers, racewalkers, and everyone in between. It offers good information about strength training, stretching, and sports nutrition.

• *The Feeling Good Handbook* by David D. Burns, M.D. Plume, 1999. Dr. Burns is one of the originators of cognitive therapy, a clinically proven, drug-free therapy for depression. This handbook features a practical, step-by-step program based on cognitive therapy that will be especially helpful for women struggling with anxiety, guilt, pessimism, procrastination, and low-self esteem.

• *Fitness Walking for Dummies* by Liz Neporent. Hungry Minds, Inc., 1999. Despite its title, this book has some smart advice for beginning walkers to high-energy walkers. It is reader-friendly and very practical.

• *For Her Own Good* by Barbara Ehrenreich and Deirdre English. Anchor Books, 1978. This book provides an eye-opening look at the way woman's moods were conceptualized and treated a hundred years ago. Well-researched and written.

• *The Omega Diet* by Artemis Simopoulos, M.D., and Jo Robinson. HarperCollins, 1998. Whether you're interested in losing weight or simply achieving optimal health, this book stands out from the other popular nutrition books in terms of its scientific merits, endorsements from experts in the field, and practical advice. The book includes a 21-day weight-loss plan that will help you lose weight and *improve* your health. An excellent weight-loss companion to the LEVITY program.

• *The Promise of Sleep* by William C. Dement, M.D., Ph.D. Dell, 1999. This book will help you understand more about the biology of sleep, including how sleep helps you heal and influences your mood. Dr. Dement, founder and director of the Stanford Research Center, shares four decades of research and clinical experience.

• *Strong Women Stay Young* by Miriam E. Nelson, Ph.D. Bantam Books, 1998. In addition to exercising to boost your mood, you may have time to engage in strength training to build your bones and preserve lean muscle. This book is aimed at older women but has good advice for women of all ages.

- *Winter Blues* by Norman Rosenthal, M.D. Guilford Press, 1998. Dr. Rosenthal, senior researcher at the National Institutes of Health and clinical professor of psychiatry at Georgetown University in Washington, D.C., led the team that first described seasonal affective disorder. This revised and updated version of his book explains the biology of SAD and how to overcome it. This book will prove helpful for women who experience the seasonal Body Blues.

- *A Woman's Guide to Sleep* by Joyce A. Walsleben, Ph.D. Times Books, 2000. This book focuses on women's unique sleep problems, including difficulties linked with hormones and family roles.

- *Women's Moods* by Deborah Sichel, M.D., and Jeanne Driscoll. Quill, 2000. This is one of the few books on depression that focuses on women's unique biology. Especially helpful for women with mood problems linked with reproductive events such as PMS and pregnancy.

The following is the complete text of the LEVITY study as it appeared in the journal *Women and Health*.

The Effects of a Multi-Modal Intervention Trial of Light, Exercise, and Vitamins on Women's Mood

Marie-Annette Brown, PhD, FNP, FAAN
Jamie Goldstein-Shirley, MSN, RN
Jo Robinson
Susan Casey, PhC, MN, RN

ABSTRACT. The purpose of this study was to test the efficacy of a tri-modal intervention (LEVITY) to improve women's mood. This eight-week randomized experiment with a placebo-control group targeted women with symptoms of mild to moderate depression. Women in the intervention group were instructed to take a brisk 20-minute outdoor walk at target heart rate of 60% of maximum heart rate, to increase light exposure throughout the day and to take a specific vitamin regimen. Women in the control group took a daily placebo vitamin. The sample consisted of 112 women ages 19-78 who reported mild to moderate depressive symptoms. They were in otherwise good health and were not currently taking any mood-altering medication. Pre-and post-intervention assessment utilized five measures of mood: Center for Epidemiology Studies Depression Scale, Profile of Mood States, Depression-Happi-

Marie-Annette Brown, Jamie Goldstein-Shirley, and Susan Casey are affiliated with the University of Washington, Seattle, WA. Jo Robinson was study volunteer.

Address correspondence to: Marie Annette Brown, PhD, FNP, University of Washington, Box 357262, Seattle, WA 98195.

This research was supported in part by grants from The Center for Women's Research at the University of Washington (supported by National Institute for Nursing Research, NIH, grant number: P30-NR04001) and Psi Chapter of Sigma Theta Tau, Seattle, WA, a chapter of Sigma Theta Tau International, Indianapolis, IN. The vitamins and placebos used in the study were supplied by Designing Health, Valencia, CA. The authors gratefully acknowledge the important contributions of the research assistants: Crista Langston, ARNP, Kathy Pearce, ARNP, Vernetta Stewart, ARNP and Ann Frolich, ARNP.

Women & Health, Vol. 34(3) 2001
2001 by The Haworth Press, Inc. All rights reserved.

172

ness Scale, Rosenberg Self-Esteem Scale, and the General Well-Being Schedule. Analysis of covariance indicated that the intervention was effective in improving women's overall mood, self-esteem, and general sense of well-being and in decreasing symptoms on two measures of depression. Of particular note, the data from all five outcome measures supported the efficacy of the intervention. In addition, a high level of adherence to the intervention protocol was observed with two-thirds of the women reporting 100% adherence. Study implications suggest that this type of intervention may provide an effective, clinically manageable therapy for mild-to-moderately depressed women who prefer a self-directed approach or who have difficulties with the cost or side-effects of medication or psychotherapy. *[Article copies available for a fee from The Haworth Document Delivery Service: 1-800-342-9678. E-mail address: <getinfo@haworthpressinc.com> Website: <http://www.HaworthPress.com> 2001 by The Haworth Press, Inc. All rights reserved.]*

KEYWORDS. Depression, subsyndromal depression, depression-atypical symptoms, vitamins, exercise, light, women, lifestyle change, alternative therapies, CES-D, POMS

INTRODUCTION

Epidemiological surveys consistently show that after adolescence, girls and women are twice as likely as are boys and men to be diagnosed with depression (Williams et al. 1995). This is true both for major depression and milder forms such as dysthymic disorder, minor depression, seasonal affective disorder (SAD), and subsyndromal depression (SSD) (Olfson et al. 1996).

Gender differences are also apparent in the manifestation of depression (Kornstein 1997). For example, women are more likely to present with vegetative or atypical symptoms such as fatigue, increased appetite, sleepiness, and weight gain, while men are more likely to present with "more typical" symptoms such as decreased appetite, insomnia, and weight loss (Frank, Carpenter, and Kupfer 1988; Young et al. 1990). Women are more likely than men to have a seasonal pattern to their depression (Lee and Chan 1998). Comorbidity is also seen more often in depressed women than in depressed men (Blazer et al. 1994; Regier, Burke, and Burke 1990). In particular, women are more likely to experience anxiety and eating disorders along with a depressed mood. Finally, several studies have shown that women may have longer episodes of depression and may be at greater risk of having a "chronic and recurrent course of illness" (Kornstein 1997, 13).

Gender may also be relevant when considering the mode of therapy, with non-pharmacological intervention especially well-suited for women. For example, drugs may have longer half-lives in women and result in more side effects and toxicity (Kornstein 1997). Also, the effectiveness of the medications can fluctuate with changes in hormone levels (e.g., pregnancy, menstrual cycle, oral contraceptives, and hormone replacement therapy). Women are more likely than men to employ alternatives to traditional medication, such as vitamins, homeopathy, and yoga (Beal 1998). In one study, women expressed a clear preference for "general psycho-educational classes about health and stress" and "less interest in group therapy and medication" (Alvidrez and Azocar 1999, 340). Despite this, female gender is a positive predictor of antidepressant use with depressed women as much as 55 percent more likely than depressed men to be prescribed antidepressant medications (Simoni-Wastila 1998).

Lifestyle interventions offer possible alternative or complementary strategies for relieving depression. Three of the most promising–exercise, increased light exposure, and specific vitamins–were selected for this study. The extensive literature on exercise suggests that exercise can have a significant antidepressant effect in mild to moderate forms of depressive illness in both men and women (Fox 1999). Blumenthal et al. (1999) determined that supervised aerobic exercise was just as effective in treating older patients with major depression as the antidepressant Sertraline. This medication is one of the newer selective serotonin reuptake inhibitors widely prescribed for the treatment of depression, which further underscores the antidepressant potential of exercise.

Exercise may have added value for women because the relationship between mood and exercise appears stronger in women than in men (Stephens 1988). Exercise may also relieve physical and emotional symptoms associated with late luteal phase dysphoria (Hightower 1997) and menopause (Slaven and Lee 1997), two conditions unique to women.

Moderate exercise has been shown to be more effective than vigorous exercise in decreasing the anxiety and stress components of depression. In a 1989 randomized, controlled trial, walking at a moderate pace for 20 minutes a day at 60% maximum heart rate was more effective in enhancing overall mood and reducing stress than more rigorous and sustained exercise at a higher heart rate. In fact, the participants who were assigned to the more vigorous program registered an *increase* in overall stress (Moses et al. 1989).

High-intensity artificial light was first identified as a treatment for seasonal depression in 1985 by Rosenthal et al. Since then, it has also proven effective in treating non-seasonal depression (Kripke et al. 1992; Beauchemin and Hays 1997; Kripke 1998), premenstrual tension (Parry et al. 1993; Lam et al. 1999), and eating disorders (Lam et al. 1994). Light therapy also has the potential to reduce common symptoms of atypical depression, like increased appetite and carbohydrate cravings (Krauchi, Wirz-Justice, and Graw 1990).

New research indicates that increased exposure to natural light may have an antidepressant effect similar to high-intensity artificial light, especially for symptoms of atypical depression. A San Diego survey determined that those adults who spent the most time out-of-doors had the fewest number of symptoms of atypical depression (Espiritu et al. 1994). In a study conducted in Finland and Sweden, "the amount of light and the length of the day as measured by monthly global radiation totals" was found to be the best single predictor of general well-being (Molin et al. 1996). A 1997 London survey of healthy women without SAD found a strong correlation between mood and outdoor light levels. Indeed, mood was more highly correlated with outdoor light levels than with the phase of a woman's menstrual cycle (Einon 1997). In a controlled trial of women with SAD, one hour of natural outdoor light had a significant antidepressant response and was as effective in treating SAD as a 2500 lux high intensity light (Wirz-Justice et al. 1996).

Certain vitamins have proven effective to enhance mood in women. In 1990, a group of female and male volunteers in a double blind cross-over trial were treated with 100 mcg of selenium and showed a significant improvement on the Profile of Mood States (POMS) in 2.5 weeks (Benton and Cook 1990). In a placebo-controlled, double-blind study, women, but not men, who took 50 milligrams of thiamine for 2 months became more clear-headed, composed and energetic (Benton, Griffiths, and Haller 1997). Vitamin D supplements have shown a rapid antidepressant effect during the winter months when sun exposure, and therefore body stores of vitamin D, are most likely to be low (Lansdowne and Provost 1998). Other vitamins with demonstrated potential for mood-enhancing effects in women are folic acid (Alpert and Fava 1997), pyridoxine and riboflavin (Benton, Fordy, and Haller 1995).

The purpose of this study was to test the efficacy of a tri-modal intervention of moderate intensity exercise, increased exposure to natural light and a specific vitamin regimen using a randomized experiment with a placebo control group. The following three rationale supported our use of a tri-modal intervention. Combining the three modalities may result in greater relief of depressive symptoms in a given individual. In the Partonen et al. study (1998), the people who took part in fitness training under bright lighting conditions experienced greater relief from both typical and atypical symptoms of depression than those who participated in the same exercise program under normal lighting conditions. Additionally, an intervention that combines several elements might influence a broader range of symptoms than a single element. For example, bright light has been show to deepen sleep (Campbell et al. 1993), an effect not demonstrated with vitamins. Similarly, exercise has been shown to improve self-esteem (McAuley et al. 1997), a benefit not commonly seen with bright light. Finally, the combination of three separate elements could also increase the likelihood of mood enhancement in a greater percentage of the study participants. In all the studies of the antidepressant effects of light, exercise or vitamins as single components, a substantial number of the participants have not benefited. For example, in a controlled trial of bright light by Kripke et al. (1992), one out of three people did not experience relief from their nonseasonal depression. It is possible that someone who fails to respond to one of the interventions would respond well to another, increasing the overall effectiveness of the program.

Although most studies designed to relieve depression have focused on a single modality, multi-faceted programs have been tested and shown to be effective (Fordyce 1977; Smith, Compton, and West 1995). The benefits of such an intervention, however, must be weighed against its disadvantages. Each added element increases the demands on the participants, potentially lowering adherence and making the program less enjoyable, as well as making it more time-consuming and thus costly for busy health care professionals to teach. Thus, we limited our intervention to a brisk, daily walk outdoors combined with taking vitamins, a regimen that required only twenty minutes a day, five times a week.

METHODS

Screening, Selection & Characteristics

Subjects were recruited from the greater Seattle area using a combination of media, including flyers, a radio talk show, a television news program, and newspaper announcements about the study. Special attention was given to recruiting women from communities of color by means of a focused distribution of flyers to businesses, churches and clinics.

Subjects were screened by a member of the research team using the following inclusion criteria: women over age 18; generally healthy with no significant chronic illness; not currently taking any medications which alter mood; and mood scores between 11 and 29 on the Center for Epidemiology Studies Depression Scale (CES-D) (Locke and Putnam 1971). A literature review suggested that this range of CESD scores would be likely to capture women with the presence of mild to moderate depressive symptoms and eliminate women with severe symptomatology or clinical depression. This range of scores also reflects the generally accepted cutoff of 16 (in a possible range of 0-60) to indicate the presence of some depressive symptomatology and the analysis of researchers who used the CES-D concurrently with a diagnostic clinical interview for depression (Weissman et al. 1997; Schulberg et al. 1985). Exclusion criteria included current daily use of high doses of specified vitamins; aerobic exercise three or more times per week; physical disability that does not allow daily brisk walking; and regular participation in life activities which occur outdoors and exceed one hour a day (e.g., employment as a gardener). Acutely depressed respondents were offered a crisis hotline number. Women whose depression scores were above the cut-off were referred to their primary care provider and encouraged to seek care for their distress.

Four hundred ninety-one women volunteered and 146 met the inclusion criteria. These 146 potential participants were mailed a consent form that included the following: a study description, the potential risks and benefits, and the possibility of receiving placebo vitamins. Of the 125 women who returned these forms, 112 women attended the first two-hour orientation session, yielding an accrual rate of 77%.

Upon arrival at the orientation session, the women completed the Time 1 questionnaires and were then randomized into two groups. To insure the integrity of the randomization process, a consulting statistician who was not a member of the research team designed and implemented the allocation procedures. One group received the entire tri-modal intervention; the other received only placebo vitamins. Because of the recruitment process, which included media discussions of the intervention program, many of the women were aware that we were interested in three particular aspects of lifestyle change. However, in the randomization process, investigators were purposefully vague about the number and nature of the groups. All participants understood that 50% of them would be given placebo vitamins. The placebo and active vitamins were identical in appearance and the bottles labeled only with a code number.

There were no statistical differences between the two groups in the demographic characteristics (See Table 1). They were generally white, college-educated, employed, middle-class women; 43% of the women reported a family income of less than $40,000, 10% reported trade or high school education, 11% were from communities of color, and 51% worked part-time or less. Their average age was 43, the age range from 19-78, with 14% under 30 and 27% over 50 years of age.

TABLE 1. Demographic Characteristics*

Characteristic	Treatment Group n = 53	Control Group n = 51
Age:		
Minimum	19	22
Maximum	78	62
Mean	43.7	41.9
Employment Status:		
Employed Full-time	27 (51%)	25 (49%)
Employed Part-time	18 (34%)	15 (29%)
Homemaker	3 (6%)	8 (16%)
Student or Other	5 (9%)	3 (6%)
Family Income:		
Under $20,000	12 (22%)	9 (18%)
$20,000-39,000	9 (18%)	12 (24%)
$40,000-79,000	21 (40%)	20 (39%)
Over $80,000	5 (9%)	5 (10%)
Declined to Answer	6 (11%)	5 (10%)
Number of Children:		
No children	22 (42%)	19 (37%)
One child	9 (17%)	9 (18%)
Two children	14 (26%)	19 (37%)
Three or more children	8 (15%)	4 (8%)
Education:		
High school or equiv	3 (6%)	2 (4%)
Some college or trade/technical school	21 (40%)	13 (25%)
Baccalaureate degree	18 (34%)	21 (41%)
Graduate school	11 (21%)	15 (29%)
Ethnicity:	One missing	
White	46 (87%)	46 (90%)
Of Color	6 (11%)	5 (10%)

* There were no statistically significant differences between the two groups on these reported characteristics.

Procedures

All the procedures and interventions in this study were approved by the human subjects committee prior to beginning the study. The intervention group was provided with a one-hour educational session about the mood-enhancing benefits of exercise, light and vitamins. The participants were instructed to walk outside during daylight hours for 20 minutes, 5 days each week, with a target heart rate of 60% of their maximum heart rate. In addition, they were asked to utilize strategies learned in the informational session to maximize their exposure to commonly available indoor and outdoor light in all aspects of their life. No high-intensity light boxes were used in this study. Finally, they were provided with a daily vitamin tablet that contained: thiamine (B1) 50 mg, pyroxidine (B6) 50 mg, riboflavin (B2) 50 mg, folic acid 400 mcg, selenium 200 mcg and vitamin D 400 IU. This combination of supplements and these specific doses were based on randomized, controlled trials to verify their effectiveness in improving mood.

Each woman was assigned to a member of the research team who served as her "coach." The coach taught her to calculate her target heart rate (220 minus age times 0.6), take her own pulse, and determine the pace necessary to attain her target heart rate. Women were instructed to monitor their heart rate several times during their daily walk and to focus on what pace was necessary for them to achieve their target heart rate. Coaches also assisted the women to develop strategies to integrate the lifestyle changes into their daily routines. The coach contacted each woman with a brief phone call at two-week intervals to assist her to overcome barriers to adherence. This coaching was streamlined to reflect the kind of counseling currently offered by nurse practitioners in clinical settings who are helping patients implement lifestyle changes.

The control group members, by contrast, received a educational session about the mood-enhancing effects of vitamins, were given an 8-week supply of placebo vitamin tablets to take daily, and were assigned a coach. They received the same supportive coaching calls throughout the study period to assist with overcoming barriers to adherence in regular vitamin use.

At the completion of the study, the control group members were notified of their group assignment, given general information about the placebo effect, and provided with active vitamins. They were also offered the opportunity to participate in the full intervention, including 8 weeks of supportive coaching.

All of the instruments below were completed at the orientation session (Time 1) and immediately post-intervention (Time 2). In addition to the standardized instruments, information about demographics, lifestyle habits, and general health status was collected. During the course of the intervention, all participants were asked to complete a brief daily diary documenting their adherence to their group's intervention. After completing the Time 2 questionnaires, women in the intervention group participated in taped interviews to obtain qualitative data about the challenges and benefits of participation in the intervention.

Instruments

The following measures were used to assess the perceived well-being of the participants. The women were asked to consider the previous two weeks as the referent time period in responding to the questions.

Center for Epidemiology Studies Depression Scale (CES-D) (Locke and Putnam 1971) is a 20-item scale that measures current affective depression. It was designed to assess for depression in the general community, rather than differentiate among clinical populations, and has been used extensively in research (Cronbach's alpha = 0.83). The 25-item Depression-Happiness Scale (DHS) (McGreal and Joseph 1993) was developed to measure variation along the continuum from depression to happiness. By including items that assess positive mood, this scale is designed to compensate for the narrow range of mood variation described by other scales, such as the CES-D, which are designed to detect only depression (Cronbach's alpha = 0.92). The 10-item Rosenberg Self-Esteem Scale (Rosenberg 1965) measures self-esteem as a global favorable or unfavorable attitude (Cronbach's alpha = 0.86). The Profile of Mood States (POMS) (McNair, Lorr, and Droppleman 1971) is a 65-item survey divided into six factorally-derived subscales: vigor, tension, fatigue, confusion, anger, and depression (Cronbach's alpha = 0.91). The 18-item General Well-Being Schedule (GWB) (Monk 1981) is a broad indicator of psychological well-being with six subscales: anxiety, depression, general health, positive well-being, self-control, and vitality (Cronbach's alpha = 0.85). The 16-item Levity Inventory was developed by the investigators and pilot tested during this study. The scale included indicators of atypical depression, as well as other aspects of well-being, including optimism, satisfaction with physical and mental health state, and positive coping behaviors. Due to the preliminary nature of the scale, it was not analyzed as an outcome measure. However, initial performance measures were promising and correlations with the other outcome variables ranged from 0.42 to 0.57 (Cronbach's = 0.78).

Statistical Analysis

Demographic characteristics of the two groups were compared using ANOVA and t-tests. Efficacy analysis was designed to evaluate the change in scores of the major dependent variables from Time 1 to Time 2 using analysis of covariance (ANCOVA).

RESULTS

Major Dependent Variables

The ANCOVA results indicate that the intervention was effective in improving women's overall mood, self-esteem and general sense of well-being and in decreasing their depression. Despite random assignment, at Time 1 the control group reported lower mood and general well-being, greater depression, and lower self-esteem than the intervention group. Both groups improved significantly (as reflected in the paired t-tests reported in Table 2) on every dependent variable, but for all outcomes, the ANCOVA revealed that the women in the intervention group improved significantly more than their control group counterparts. All but 4 of the 53 participants in the intervention group improved or had no change in their depression scores, whereas, the participants in the control group exhibited more variability in their outcomes.

Additional analysis further illuminated the effects of the intervention on the atypical symptoms of depression. Women in the intervention group reported decreased tension and anger as measured by the POMS subscales (Table 3). The subscales of the GWB revealed that the women experienced decreased depression and increased self-control, vitality, and positive well-being (Table 4).

Further analyses were also conducted to determine whether the level of depressive symptoms was related to the degree of women's improvement in mood during the intervention. A MANCOVA was used to stratify the participants into two groups by their Time 1 CES-D score on a median split. The results of the analysis indicated that there was no significant interaction effect; thus the intervention was equally efficacious for women with varying levels of symptomatology.

TABLE 2. Total Scales Means and ANCOVA Significance (N(Control) = 51, N(Treatment) = 53)

Scale	Interpretation	Group	Time 1 Mean	SD+	Time 2 Mean	SD	Change Score Mean	SD	Paired T-test#	ANCOVA Significance*
CES-D	Higher score indicates more depression	Control	22.2	8.3	16.7	10.4	5.5	10.2	.000	.004
		Treatment	19.0	7.8	10.4	7.3	8.6	9.2	.000	
Depression-Happiness	Higher score indicates more happiness	Control	40.7	12.5	48.8	14.1	8.1	14.1	.000	.002
		Treatment	46.3	12.5	58.8	12.0	12.5	13.0	.000	
Rosenberg Self-Esteem	Higher score indicates less self-esteem	Control	22.5	4.8	20.7	5.2	1.8	4.1	.003	.003
		Treatment	20.6	4.8	17.0	4.8	3.5	4.9	.000	
General Well-Being	Higher score indicates greater sense of well-being	Control	52.9	12.8	64.3	16.8	11.4	16.6	.000	.008
		Treatment	59.3	13.2	74.3	12.1	15.0	15.4	.000	
POMS	Higher score indicates greater mood disturbance	Control	79.1	26.3	60.4	33.5	18.8	29.8	.000	.015
		Treatment	64.0	23.4	39.6	22.5	24.2	26.0	.000	

+ At Time 1, the control group scores were significantly (p > .05) worse on all scales
# Paired t-tests compare Time 2 to Time 1 scores for each group
* p-value for ANCOVA comparing post-test scores controlling for pre-test scores

TABLE 3. POMS Subscales (N(Control) = 51, N(Treatment) = 53

| | | Time 1 | | Time 2 | | ANCOVA |
Scale	Group	Mean	SD+	Mean	SD	Significance*
Vigor	Control	10.0	5.0	13.7	5.8	.066
	Treatment	12.1	5.4	16.8	6.5	NS
Tension	Control	13.9	6.0	12.0	7.2	.012
	Treatment	11.7	4.6	8.1	4.4	
Fatigue	Control	15.3	5.7	10.8	6.3	.135
	Treatment	12.0	5.9	7.7	4.9	NS
Confusion	Control	10.8	5.1	7.7	5.3	.102
	Treatment	8.6	3.6	5.4	3.2	NS
Anger	Control	19.9	9.8	12.4	9.2	.002
	Treatment	15.1	8.0	7.4	5.1	
Depression	Control	19.9	9.8	13.8	10.3	.067
	Treatment	15.1	8.0	8.5	7.7	NS

+ At Time 1, the control group scores were significantly (p > .05) worse on all scales
* p-value for ANCOVA comparing post-test scores controlling for pre-test score

TABLE 4. General Well-Being Subscales (N(Control) = 51, N(Treatment) = 53

| | | Time 1 | | Time 2 | | ANCOVA |
Scale	Group	Mean	SD+	Mean	SD	Significance*
Anxiety	Control	15.4	4.2	17.0	5.2	.200
	Treatment	17.2	4.1	18.9	3.6	NS
Depression	Control	13.1	3.2	15.2	3.3	.03
	Treatment	14.0	3.3	16.8	3.1	
Positive Well-Being	Control	8.7	2.1	10.2	3.0	.009
	Treatment	9.8	2.2	12.0	2.7	
Self-Control	Control	12.4	2.4	13.5	2.8	.006
	Treatment	12.7	2.5	14.8	2.3	
Vitality	Control	9.2	3.1	12.0	3.9	.015
	Treatment	11.1	3.6	14.3	3.3	
Health	Control	9.9	3.7	10.4	3.7	.178
	Treatment	10.4	3.1	11.5	3.0	NS

+ At Time 1, the control group scores were significantly (p > .05) worse on all scales
* p-value for ANCOVA comparing post-test scores controlling for pre-test score

Perception of Mood Improvement

At Time 2, women were asked to give a subjective overall impression of their change in mood over the 8 weeks of the project on a 7-point scale from "a lot better" to "a lot worse." In the control group, 59% reported that they had at least some improvement in mood from the beginning of the study. In contrast, 85% of the intervention group reported improved mood. Thirty-seven percent of the control group felt that their mood stayed the same over the course of the study, while only 11% of the intervention group reported this perception. Two women in each group (representing 4% of each group) reported that their mood was worse at the end of the study period. Further analysis explored the extent to which this overall subjective summary of mood change was associated with change on the five dependent variables. There was a moderate to high correlation between women's perceived change in mood and their change scores derived from the standardized instruments ($r = .54$ to $.68$, $p = .00$ for all correlations).

Adherence to the Intervention Protocol

A high level of adherence to the intervention regimen was recorded in the women's logbooks. A total adherence score was calculated as the sum of the number of occurrences of each the activities (days when walking, light exposure, or vitamin taking were reported in the women's logbooks). One hundred percent adherence was considered to be 40 occurrences of walking, 40 occurrences of light, and 56 days of vitamins totaling a score of 136 in an 8-week period. Some women did more than prescribed by the intervention (for example, walked more than 5 days per week), so achieved scores higher than 136. Almost two-thirds (64%) of the women reported 100% adherence or more. Only 2 participants fell below a threshold of 73% of the total adherence score. On what might be the most challenging portion of the intervention, the walking component, 83% of the participants were compliant at 75% or better. Cited reasons for non-adherence were temporary loss of logbook, discontinuing the vitamin due to increased appetite, and persistent fatigue.

Drop-Outs

Of the 112 women who began the intervention, only 8 failed to complete the eight-week intervention and all of the questionnaires. Five of these women were in the control group and three were in the intervention group. Two of these women were lost to follow-up. This small number does not allow for comparisons with those who completed the intervention. Two primary reasons for drop-out were: (1) a decision to seek other treatment or start anti-depressants due to increased depression, and (2) a lack of time or interest.

Evidence of Minimal Cross-Over

Because the three modalities used in the intervention were discussed in media interviews by which participants were recruited, we were concerned that this awareness would prompt the control group to independently initiate behavior changes similar to the intervention protocol. At Time 2, questions were included in the questionnaire to determine the participants' exposure to light and participation in exercise. We asked participants about their light exposure prior to and during the project. Over 94% of the women reported that they usually decreased their outdoor light exposure in the winter months of the study period compared to the spring and summer. When the control group was asked about their outdoor light exposure during the project, 86% noted that they had similar or less exposure to outdoor light than in previous years. Similarly, 75% did not increase in their indoor light exposure. By contrast, the intervention group claimed significantly higher indoor and outdoor light exposure. Only 4% reported that their outdoor light exposure was similar or less than previous years. Seventy percent of the intervention group had increased their indoor light exposure during the study period. These data suggest that the majority of the control group did not change their light exposure as a result of the information they gleaned from the recruitment process.

Data about the control group's members' participation in moderate to vigorous exercise yielded similarly low levels. Only 12% of the control group had exercised to the level of the intervention (3-5 times per week) in the prior two weeks. The other 88% denied such physical activity.

Side Effects of Vitamins

Some participants in both the control (14%, n = 7) and intervention groups (30%, n = 16) reported a single minor side effects from the vitamins, such as bright yellow urine, gastrointestinal symptoms, sleep disturbances, and skin reactions.

DISCUSSION

These study findings suggest that a program of moderate-intensity walking, increased light exposure, and selected vitamins can improve women's mood. The high level of adherence to the intervention suggests that women could comfortably incorporate this tri-modal program into their daily lives. These findings extend the work of other studies that have demonstrated the positive influence of each independent component (light, exercise, and vitamins) on mood (Kripke 1998; Wirz-Justice et al. 1996; Blumenthal et al. 1999; Moses et al. 1989; Benton, Fordy, and Haller 1995).

Women in the intervention group improved significantly compared to those in the control group on all five dependent variables that measured mood and well-being. Not only did their depression scores decrease, they also reported greater self-esteem, improved general well-being, and greater happiness.

We were particularly interested in determining whether the intervention addressed symptoms more prevalent in women than men, such as anxiety and fatigue. The subscales of the POMS showed that the women in the intervention group experienced a significant decrease in anger and tension. Meanwhile their vitality improved, as measured by the GWB subscales.

Study findings suggest that the tri-modal intervention may also relieve seasonal mood swings that are more common in women than men. The study took place from October into December, a time of increasing rainfall in the Pacific Northwest. (There were 9 days of rain in the first four weeks of the study and 17 days in the second four weeks.) Thus the women were exposed to both cloudier weather and declining hours of daylight, conditions known to trigger seasonal decreases in mood. Nonetheless, the women in the intervention group experienced a significant improvement in mood.

Support for the idea that a tri-modal lifestyle intervention might prove more broadly effective than a solitary intervention comes from a comparison of our results with the results of Moses et al. (1989), that used brisk walking at 60% of maximum heart rate for 20 minutes as the only intervention and used the POMS as one outcome measure. Moses et al. observed improvement on one subscale of the POMS (tension) while the LEVITY participants improved on two (tension and anger). Moses et al. reported one non-significant trend in the confusion subscale, whereas this study found non-significant trends in both the depression and vigor scales. LEVITY participants also improved on the total POMS. (Moses et al. presented results on the subscales only.) This broader improvement shown by combining light and vitamins with moderate-intensity exercise suggests that multi-modal interventions warrant further study.

Our ability to test our supposition that this tri-modal intervention would be effective for a larger percentage of participants than single-modality interventions was limited. To explore this supposition, we calculated the number of participants in the intervention group whose improvement in mood, as measured by the CES-D, exceeded that of the mean change score of the control group (>5.5 points). Nearly two-thirds (63%) of the intervention group had improvement in their CES-D scores greater than 5.5 points from Time 1 to Time 2.

RESPONSE OF THE CONTROL GROUP

It is important to discuss the significant improvement in mood that occurred in members of the control group. To isolate the measurement of the effects of the intervention protocol (light, exercise and vitamins), the control group was exposed to potentially mood enhancing elements that mimicked those received by the intervention group. These included placebo vitamins, attention from coaches and new information about depression. The combination of these aspects could account for the observed improvement in mood in the control group.

Another explanation for the improvement in the control group is regression toward the mean. Despite random assignment after initial data collection and comparable demographic characteristics, there was a significant difference between the two groups on the dependent variables upon entry into the study (see Table 2). Strict attention to randomization procedures does not guarantee equal/comparable groups because of the variability within the larger sample. Because the control group was more depressed and reported more negative well-being scores at Time 1, it was likely that their scores would improve, moving closer to population averages at Time 2. Therefore, the ANCOVA analysis was used to control for this difference.

These methodological and statistical considerations, however, should be distinguished from concerns about unintended design contamination (self-initiated exercise and light program). While the control group participants were aware of the tri-modal nature of the intervention, the data reported earlier demonstrates that there was minimal cross-over.

STUDY LIMITATIONS

Study results need to be considered in light of the limitations inherent in the design. The self-selection bias of women volunteering for the study could have yielded women in the action-oriented phase of behavior change as described by Prochaska et al. (1994), a stage characterized by increased motivation and commitment. A woman presenting symptoms of depression to her health care provider may not be as motivated. Also, the relationship that developed between the coaches and participants might have increased the participants' motivation, or elicited socially desirable responses. These factors could influence the effectiveness of the intervention in actual clinical application.

Additionally, the study participants do not reflect the race and class diversity in the American population. They were, in general, white, middle-class, and well-educated. Because of their privileged status, they were more likely to have flexibility in working arrangements, a safe walking environment, and access to childcare. This intervention warrants further testing in a broader population, including different ages, partner status, ethnicity, and class.

Although other research documents the effectiveness of each individual component of this intervention, this study does not allow direct comparisons between the effects of light, exercise, vitamins, and the combination of all three components. The next step in this program of research will include design aspects that allow for the separation of the effects of each component. The design could also be enhanced by a larger, more diverse sample and by selecting participants using diagnostic tools (such as the HAM-D).

The results of this study offer preliminary support for the use of this tri-modal intervention that would offer primary care practitioners a low cost, effective treatment for mild depression as an alternative to the use of psychotropic medications and referrals for psychotherapy. The costs and side-effects of these standard therapies had led the women in our study to seek another option. This intervention is simple enough that the instructions can be conveyed in a standard 15-minute appointment and accomplished without direct supervision. Additionally, it would be feasible for women to independently re-initiate the program should they experience recurring or chronic depression. Indeed, our participants were able to easily incorporate all components into their daily lives and maintain a commitment to the program. They reported satisfaction in knowing that their improved mood was due to their own activities, not a prescribed medication. As one participant noted: "I found there was something I could do that was within my own control. I didn't have to go to the doctor to get a prescription. It is such a helpless feeling to not know how to change your moods."

REFERENCES

Alpert, J. E., and M. Fava. 1977. Nutrition and depression: The role of folate. *Nutrition Reviews* 55(5):145-49.

Alvidrez, J., and F. Azocar. 1999. Distressed women's clinic patients: Preferences for mental health treatments and perceived obstacles. *Gen Hosp Psychiatry* 21(5): 340-47.

Beal, M. W. 1998. Women's use of complementary and alternative therapies in reproductive health care. *J Nurse Midwifery* 43(3): 224-34.

Beauchemin, K.M., and P. Hays. 1997. Phototherapy is a useful adjunct in the treatment of depressed in-patients. *Acta Psychiatr Scand* 95:424-27.

Benton, D., and R. Cook. 1990. Selenium supplementation improves mood in a double-blind crossover trial. *Psychopharmacology* 102:549-50.

Benton, D., J. Fordy, and J. Haller. 1995. The impact of long-term vitamin supplementation on cognitive functioning. *Psychopharmacology (Berl)* 117:298-305.

Benton, D., R. Griffiths, and J. Haller. 1997. Thiamine supplementation, mood, and cognitive functioning. *Psychopharmacology* 129:66-71.

Blazer, D.G., R.C. Kessler, K.A. McGonagle, and M.S. Swartz. 1994. The prevalence and distribution of major depression in a national community sample: the National Comorbidity Survey. *Am J Psychiatry* 151:979-86.

Blumenthal, J.A., M.A. Babyak, K.A. Moore, W.E. Craighead, S. Herman, P. Khatri, R. Waugh, M.A. Napolitano, L.M., Forman, M. Appelbaum, P.M. Doraiswamy, and K.R. Krishnan. 1999. Effects of exercise training in older patients with major depression. *Arch Intern Med* 159(19):2349-56.

Campbell, S. S., D. Dawson, and M.W. Anderson. 1993. Alleviation of sleep maintenance insomnia with timed exposure to bright light. *J Am Geriatr Soc* 41(8):829-36.

Einon, D. 1997. The influence of ambient light and menstrual status on the moods of a nonclinical population of young women. *Psychosomatic Medicine* 59:616-19.

Espiritu, R. C., D. F. Kripke, S. Ancoli-Israel, M. A. Mowen, W. J. Mason, R. L. Fell, M. R. Klauber, and O. J. Kaplan. 1994. Low illumination experienced by San Diego adults: association with atypical depressive symptoms. *Biol Psychiatry* 35:403-07.

Fordyce, M. W. 1977. Development of a program to increase personal happiness. *J Counseling Psychology* 24:511-21.

Fox, K. R. 1999. The influence of physical activity on mental well-being. *Public Health Nutr* 2: 411-18.

Frank, E., L. L. Carpenter, and D. J. Kupfer. 1988. Sex differences in recurrent depression: are there any that are significant? *Am J Psychiatry* 145:41-45.

Hightower, M. 1997. Effects of exercise participation on menstrual pain and symptoms. *Women Health* 26(4):15-27.

Kornstein, S. G. 1997. Gender differences in depression: implications for treatment. *J Clin Psychiatry* 58(Suppl 15):12-18.

Kripke, D. F. 1998. Light treatment for nonseasonal depression: speed, efficacy, and combined treatment. *J Affect Disord* 49(2):109-17.

Kripke, D.F., D.J. Mullaney, M.R. Klauber, S.C. Risch, and J.C. Gillin. 1992. Controlled trial of bright light for nonseasonal major depressive disorders. *Biol Psychiatry* 31(2):119-34.

Krauchi, K., A. Wirz-Justice, and P. Graw. 1990. The relationship of affective state to dietary preference: winter depression and light therapy as a model. *J Affect Disord* 20:43-53.

Lam, R. W., D. Carter, S. Misri, A. J. Kuan, L. N. Yatham, and A. P. Zis. 1999. A controlled study of light therapy in women with late luteal phase dysphoric disorder. *Psychiatry Res* 86(3):185-92.

Lam, R. W., E. Goldner, L. Solyom, and R. A. Remick. 1994. A controlled study of light therapy for bulimia nervosa. *Am J. Psychiatry* 151:744-750.

Lansdowne, A. T., and S. C. Provost. 1998. Vitamin D3 enhances mood in healthy subjects during winter. *Psychopharmacology (Berl)* 135:319-23.

Lee, T. M., and C. C. Chan. 1998. Vulnerability by sex to seasonal affective disorder. *Percept Mot Skills* 87:1120-22.

Locke, B. A. and P. Putman. 1971. *Center for Epidemiological Studies Depression Scale.* Washington, DC: Epidemiology and Psychopathology Research Branch, Public Health Service, National Institute of Mental Health.

McAuley, E., S. L. Mihalko, and S. M. Bane. 1997. Exercise and self-esteem in middle-aged adults: Multidimensional relationships and physical fitness and self-efficacy influences. *J Behav Med* 20: 67-83.

McGreal, R., and S. Joseph. 1993. The Depression-Happiness Scale. *Psychological Reports* 73: 1279-82.

McNair, D. M., M. Lorr, and L. F. Droppleman. 1971. *Manual for the Profile of Mood States.* San Diego, CA: Educational and Industrial Testing Service.

Molin, J., E. Mellerup, T. Bolwig, T. Scheike, and H. Dam. 1996. The influence of climate on development of winter depression. *J Affective Disorders* 37:151-55.

Monk, M. 1981. Blood pressure awareness and psychological well-being in the Health and Nutrition Examination Survey. *Clinical Investigations in Medicine* 4:183-89.

Moses, J., A. Steptoe, A. Mathews, and S. Edwards. 1989. The effects of exercise training on mental well-being in the normal population: A controlled trial. *J Psychosom Res* 33:47-61.

Olfson, M., E. Broadhead, M. M. Weissman, A. C. Leon, L. Farber, C. Hoven, and R. Kathol. 1996. Subthreshold psychiatric symptoms in a primary care group practice. *Arch Gen Psychiatry* 53:880-6.

Parry, B.L., A. M. Mahan, N. Mostofi, M. R. Klauber, G.S. Lew, and J.C. Gillin. 1993. Light therapy of late luteal phase dysphoric disorder: an extended study. *Am J Psychiatry* 150(9):1417-19.

Partonen, T., S. Leppamaki, J. Hurme, and J. Lonnqvist. 1998. Randomized trial of physical exercise alone or combined with bright light on mood and health-related quality of life. *Psychol Med* 28:1359-64.

Prochaska, J. O., J. C. Norcross, and C. C. DiClemente. 1994. *Changing for Good.* NY: Avon Books.

Regier, D. A., J. D. Burke, and K. C. Burke. 1990. Comorbidity of affective and anxiety disorders in the NIMH Epidemiologic Catchment Area Program. In J. D. Maser and C. R. Cloninger, eds., *Comorbidity of Mood and Anxiety Disorders.* Washington, DC: American Psychiatric Press. pp. 113-122.

Rejeski, W. J., L. R. Brawley, and S. A. Shumaker. 1996. Physical activity and health-related quality of life. *Exerc Sport Sci Rev* 24:71-108.

Rosenberg, M. 1965. *Society and the adolescent self-image.* Princeton, NJ: Princeton University Press.

Rosenthal, N. E., D. A. Sack, C. J. Carpenter, B. L. Parry, W. B. Mendelson, and T. A. Wehr. 1985. Antidepressant effects of light in seasonal affective disorder. *Am J Psychiatry* 142(2):163-70.

Schulberg H. C., M. Saul, M. McClelland, M. Ganguli, W. Christy, and R. Frank. 1985. Assessing depression in primary medical and psychiatric practices. *Arch Gen Psychiatry* 42:1164-70.

Simoni-Wastila, L. 1998. Gender and psychotropic drug use. *Med Care* 36(1):88-94.

Slaven, L., and C. Lee. 1997. Mood and symptom reporting among middle-aged women: The relationship between menopausal status, hormone replacement therapy, and exercise participation. *Health Psychology* 16:203-08.

Smith, P. W., W. C. Compton, and W. B. West. 1995. Meditation as an adjunct to a happiness enhancement program. *J Clinical Psychology* 51:269-73.

Stephens, T. 1988. Physical activity and mental health in the United States and Canada: Evidence from four population surveys. *Preventive Medicine* 17:33-47.

Weissman, M. M., D. Sholomskas, M. Pottenger, B. A. Prusoff, and B. Z. Locke. 1977. Assessing depressive symptoms in five psychiatric populations: A validation study. *Am J Epidemiology* 106(3): 203-13.

Williams, J. B., R. L. Spitzer, M. Linzer, K. Kroenke, S. R. Hahn, F. V. deGruy, and A. Lazev. 1995. Gender differences in depression in primary care. *Am J Obstet Gynecol* 173:654-59.

Wirz-Justice, A., P. Graw, K. Krauchi, A. Sarrafzadeh, J. English, J. Arendt, and L. Sand. 1996. Natural light treatment of seasonal affective disorder. *J Affective Disorders* 37:109-20.

Young, M. A., W. A. Scheftner, J. Fawcett, and G. L. Klerman. 1990. Gender differences in the clinical features of unipolar major depressive disorder. *J Nerv Ment Dis* 178:200-03.

Notes and References

Chapter 1

1. There is a lack of consensus about what to call these particular symptoms. They have been called *anxious somatic depressive* symptoms, *atypical depressive* symptoms, *reverse vegetative* symptoms, *reverse neurovegetative* symptoms, and *atypical symptoms of depression*. In some European countries, they are still referred to as *neurotic depressive* symptoms, a term that has fallen out of favor in many parts of the world. To make matters even more confusing, all of these various terms have slightly different definitions. For example, one diagnostic criterion will require that a person experience "leaden paralysis" (a feeling of heaviness in the limbs) while another will emphasize emotional reactivity and sensitivity to rejection.

2. Schatzberg, A. F. (2000). New indications for antidepressants. *J. Clin. Psychiatry* 61 (11 Suppl): 9–17.

3. Biver, F., F. Lotstra, M. Monclus, D. Wikler, P. Damhaut, J. Mendlewicz, and S. Goldman (1996). Sex difference in 5ht2 [serotonin] receptor in the living human brain. *Neurosci. Lett.* 204 (1–2): 25–8.

4. There are hundreds of animal and human studies that have contributed to this discovery. A few are cited below.

   Shepherd, J. E. (2001). Effects of estrogen on cognition, mood, and degenerative brain diseases. *J. Am. Pharm. Assoc.* (Wash) 41 (2): 221–8.

   Heninger, George R. (1997). Serotonin, sex, and psychiatric illness. *Proc. Natl. Acad. Sci.* 94: 4823–4.

   Lippert, T. H., M. Filshie, A. O. Muck, H. Seeger, and M. Zwirner (1996). Serotonin metabolite excretion after postmenopausal estradiol therapy. *Maturitas* 24 (1–2): 37–41.

   Fink, G., B. E. Sumner, R. Rosie, O. Grace, and J. P. Quinn (1996). Estrogen control of central neurotransmission: Effect on mood, mental state, and memory. *Cell. Mol. Neurobiol.* 16 (3): 325–44.

Panay, N., and J. W. Studd (1998). The psychotherapeutic effects of estrogens. *Gynecol. Endocrinol.* 12 (5): 353–65.

5. Nishizawa, S., C. Benkelfat, S. N. Young, M. Leyton, S. Mzengeza, C. de Montigny, P. Blier, and M. Diksic (1997). Differences between males and females in rates of serotonin synthesis in human brain. *Proc. Natl. Acad. Sci. U S A* 94 (10): 5308–13.

6. This particular test was the "Community Epidemiological Study–Depression" or CES–D. It is designed to screen the general population for signs of depression.

7. We chose *Women and Health* because it is an interdisciplinary journal read by psychologists, social workers, and people in women's studies as well as nurses and doctors.

8. At the present time, no one has surveyed large groups of women for these specific symptoms, so it is not possible to make a more accurate estimate. But my "one out of four" is probably too conservative. For example, 60 percent of all menstruating women have mild to severe symptoms of PMS. (According to the U.S. 2000 census, approximately 60 million U.S. women are between the ages of 15 and 44—the time of life when they most likely are vulnerable to PMS.) Another high-risk zone for the Body Blues is perimenopause, the 5 to 10 years leading up to menopause. There are 20 million women in this transition zone. Approximately 8 million American women have moderate levels of winter depression, another manifestation of the syndrome. Finally, fatigue, overeating, and sleep problems are endemic among women at any time of the month or year.

Chapter 2

1. Guicheney, P., D. Leger, et al. (1988). Platelet serotonin content and plasma tryptophan in peri- and postmenopausal women: Variations with plasma oestrogen levels and depressive symptoms. *Eur. J. Clin. Invest.* 18 (3): 297–304.

2. Fink, G., B. E. Sumner, et al. (1996). Estrogen control of central neurotransmission: Effect on mood, mental state, and memory. *Cell. Mol. Neurobiol.* 16 (3): 325–44.

3. Shepherd, J. E. (2001). Effects of estrogen on cognition, mood, and degenerative brain diseases. *J. Am. Pharm. Assoc.* (Wash) 41 (2): 221–8.

4. Donohoe, R. T., and D. Benton (1999). Cognitive functioning is susceptible to the level of blood glucose. *Psychopharmacology* (Berl) 145 (4): 378–85.

5. McEwen, B. S., and C. S. Woolley (1994). Estradiol and progesterone regulate neuronal structure and synaptic connectivity in adult as well as developing brain. *Exp. Gerontol.* 29 (3–4): 431–6.

6. Toran-Allerand, C. D., M. Singh, et al. (1999). Novel mechanisms of estrogen action in the brain: New players in an old story. *Front. Neuroendocrinol.* 20 (2): 97–121.

7. Warga, Claire (1999). *Menopause and the Mind.* New York: Simon & Schuster.

8. Sherwin, B. B. (1999). Can estrogen keep you smart? Evidence from clinical studies. *J. Psychiatry Neurosci.* 24 (4): 315–21.

9. Jennings, P. J., J. S. Janowsky, et al. (1998). Estrogen and sequential movement. *Behav. Neurosci.* 112 (1): 154–9.

10. For convenience sake, estradiol and progesterone have been drawn to the same scale. In reality, progesterone is measured in nanograms and estradiol in picograms. If they were represented at their true levels, they would not fit on the same chart.

11. Sherwin, B. B. (1999). Progestogens used in menopause: Side effects, mood, and quality of life. *J. Reprod. Med.* 44 (2 Suppl): 227–32.

12. Brackley, K. J., M. M. Ramsay, et al. (1999). The effect of the menstrual cycle on human cerebral blood flow: Studies using Doppler ultrasound. *Ultrasound Obstet. Gynecol.* 14 (1): 52–7.

13. McEwen, B. S. (1998). Multiple ovarian hormone effects on brain structure and function. *J. Gend. Specif. Med.* 1 (1): 33–41.

14. Arafat, E. S., J. T. Hargrove, et al. (1988). Sedative and hypnotic effects of oral administration of micronized progesterone may be mediated through its metabolites. *Am. J. Obstet. Gynecol.* 159 (5): 1203–9.

15. Manber, R., and R. Armitage (1999). Sex, steroids, and sleep: A review. *Sleep* 22 (5): 540–55.

16. Meston, C. M., and P. F. Frohlich (2000). The neurobiology of sexual function. *Arch. Gen. Psychiatry* 57 (11): 1012–30.

17. Laumann, E. O., J. H. Gagnon, R. T. Michael, and S. Michaels (1994). *The Social Organization of Sexuality.* Chicago: University of Chicago Press.

18. Sherwin, B. B., M. M. Gelfand, et al. (1985). Androgen enhances sexual motivation in females: A prospective, crossover study of sex steroid administration in the surgical menopause. *Psychosom. Med.* 47 (4): 339–51.

19. Davis, S. R., and J. Tran (2001). Testosterone influences libido and well-being in women. *Trends Endocrinol. Metab.* 12 (1): 33–7.

20. Tuiten, A., J. Van Honk, et al. (2000). Time course of effects of testosterone administration on sexual arousal in women. *Arch. Gen. Psychiatry* 57 (2): 149–53; discussion 155–6.

21. Sherwin, B. B. (1988). Affective changes with estrogen and androgen replacement therapy in surgically menopausal women. *J. Affect. Disord.* 14 (2): 177–87.

22. Zumoff, B., G. W. Strain, et al. (1995). Twenty-four-hour mean plasma testosterone concentration declines with age in normal premenopausal women. *J. Clin. Endocrinol. Metab.* 80 (4): 1429–30.

23. Casson, P. R., K. E. Elkind-Hirsch, et al. (1997). Effect of postmenopausal estrogen replacement on circulating androgens. *Obstet. Gynecol.* 90 (6): 995–8.

24. Targum, S. D., K. P. Caputo, et al. (1991). Menstrual cycle phase and psychiatric admissions. *J. Affect. Disord.* 22 (1–2): 49–53.

25. Gladis, M. M., and B. T. Walsh (1987). Premenstrual exacerbation of binge eating in bulimia. *Am. J. Psychiatry* 144 (12): 1592–5.

26. Chaturvedi, S. K., P. S. Chandra, et al. (1995). Suicidal ideas during premenstrual phase. *J. Affect. Disord.* 34 (3): 193–9.

27. D'Orban, P. T., and J. Dalton (1980). Violent crime and the menstrual cycle. *Psychol. Med.* 10 (2): 353–9.

28. Sigmon, S. T., D. M. Dorhofer, et al. (2000). Psychophysiological, somatic, and affective changes across the menstrual cycle in women with panic disorder. *J. Consult. Clin. Psychol.* 68 (3): 425–31.

29. Angold, A., E. J. Costello, et al. (1999). Pubertal changes in hormone levels and depression in girls. *Psychol. Med.* 29 (5): 1043–53.

30. Hamilton, J. A., B. L. Parry, et al. (1988). The menstrual cycle in context (part 1): Affective syndromes associated with reproductive hormonal changes. *J. Clin. Psychiatry* 49 (12): 474–80.

31. Mitchell, E. S., N. F. Woods, and A. Mariella (2000). Three stages of the menopausal transition from the Seattle midlife women's health study: Toward a more precise definition. *Menopause* 7: 334–49.

32. Soares, C. N., and L. S. Cohen (2001). The perimenopause, depressive disorders, and hormonal variability. *Sao Paulo Med. J.* 119 (2): 78–83.

33. Schmidt, P. J., C. A. Roca, et al. (1997). The perimenopause and affective disorders. *Semin. Reprod. Endocrinol.* 15 (1): 91–100.

34. Carlson, L. E., and B. B. Sherwin (2000). Higher levels of plasma estradiol and testosterone in healthy elderly men compared with age-matched women may protect aspects of explicit memory. *Menopause* 7 (3): 168–77.

35. Khan, S. A., J. E. Pace, et al. (1994). Climacteric symptoms in healthy middle-aged women. *Br. J. Clin. Pract.* 48 (5): 240–2.

36. Anthony, T., and J. C. Anthony (2000). The estimated rate of depressed mood in U.S. adults: Recent evidence for a peak in later life. *J. Affect. Disord.* 60 (3): 159–71.

37. Luine, V. N., and J. C. Rhodes (1983). Gonadal hormone regulation of MAO and other enzymes in hypothalamic areas. *Neuroendocrinology* 36 (3): 235–41.

38. Wu, C. Y., T. J. Yu, et al. (2000). Age-related testosterone level changes and male andropause syndrome. *Changgeng Yi Xue Za Zhi* 23 (6): 348–53.

39. Carlson, L. E., and B. B. Sherwin (2000). Higher levels of plasma estradiol and testosterone in healthy elderly men compared with age-matched women may protect aspects of explicit memory. *Menopause* 7 (3): 168–77.

Chapter 3

1. In 2001, an intriguing study published in the *New England Journal of Medicine* brought into question the validity of the placebo effect. A review of the medical literature had shown that when the results of a study

could be measured objectively (for example, in blood tests or x-rays), people given placebos did only slightly better than those who received no treatment at all. The authors of the study suggested that the primary reason for the placebo effect was simply the natural course of the disease. They argued that many people get better over time, whether or not they get any treatment. Therefore, it may not be wishful thinking that helps people recover, it's simply the fact that a disease has run its course. But when the reviewers turned their attention to mood or pain studies, they did find an active placebo effect. Placebos may influence how we feel but have less impact on conditions that do not involve mood or pain. Hrobjartsson, A., and P. C. Gotzsche (2001). Is the placebo powerless? An analysis of clinical trials comparing placebo with no treatment. *N. Engl. J. Med.* 344 (21): 1594–602.

2. Harris, S., and B. Dawson-Hughes (1993). Seasonal mood changes in 250 normal women. *Psychiatry Res.* 49: 77–87.

3. For more test information, refer to our study on page 172 of this book.

4. To continue our subterfuge, we marked some of the bottles of placebo pills with a "1" and another with a "2" and handed them out randomly to the women in the placebo group. The women assumed that half of them were being given the "real" vitamins and the other half the placebos, when, in reality, they were all being given placebos.

5. To determine if the LEVITY program had relieved the Body Blues, we created six new subscales from the six tests we had used. There was a statistically significant difference between the treatment group and the placebo group in the Total Body Blues Scale (ANCOVA Significance p=.05), Stress (p=.009), Irritability (p=.001), Weight gain and appetite (p=.03), and Anxiety (p=.03). There was a nonsignificant trend of improvement in the Confusion (p=.14) and the Fatigue (p=.10) subscales.

6. Babyak, M., J. A. Blumenthal, et al. (2000). Exercise treatment for major depression: Maintenance of therapeutic benefit at 10 months. *Psychosom. Med.* 62 (5): 633–8.

7. As quoted in Elias, Marilyn (2001). Exercising may fight depression. *USA Today Health On-Line*, 10 January.

Chapter 4

1. Leproult, R., E. F. Colecchia, M. L'Hermite-Baleriaux, and E. Van Cauter (2001). Transition from dim to bright light in the morning induces an immediate elevation of cortisol levels. *J. Clin. Endocrinol. Metab.* 86: 151–57. (Note that the bright light creates normal daytime cortisol levels, not the higher levels associated with stress.)

2. Another common measurement for light is the *lumen*. One lumen equals the amount of light generated by a single standard candle. A foot-candle is defined as one lumen of uniform luminance over the area of 1 square foot.

3. Dr. Kripke's comment appeared in Kapla, Arline (1999). Light treatment for nonseasonal depression. *Psychiatric Times* 16 (3). Available from http://www.mhsource.com/pt/p990359.html; Internet.

4. Espiritu, R. C., D. F. Kripke, S. Ancoli-Israel, M. A. Mowen, W. J. Mason, R. L. Fell, M. R. Klauber, and O. J. Kaplan (1994). Low illumination experienced by San Diego adults: Association with atypical depressive symptoms. *Biol. Psychiatry* 35: 403–7.

5. Ibid, 406.

6. Jean-Louis, G., D. F. Kripke, S. Ancoli-Israel, M. R. Klauber, and R. S. Sepulveda (2000). Sleep duration, illumination, and activity patterns in a population sample: Effects of gender and ethnicity. *Biol. Psychiatry* 47: 921–7.

7. Einon, D. (1997). The influence of ambient light and menstrual status on the moods of a nonclinical population of young women. *Psychosom. Med.* 59: 616–9.

8. Smedh, K., O. Spigset, P. Allard, T. Mjorndal, and R. Adolfsson (1999). Platelet [3H]paroxetine and [3H]lysergic acid diethylamide binding in seasonal affective disorder and the effect of bright light therapy. *Biol. Psychiatry* 45: 464–70.

9. Ruhrmann, S., S. Kasper, B. Hawellek, B. Martinez, G. Hoflich, T. Nickelsen, and H. J. Moller (1998). Effects of fluoxetine versus bright light in the treatment of seasonal affective disorder. *Psychol. Med.* 28: 923–33.

10. Kripke, D. F., D. J. Mullaney, M. R. Klauber, S. C. Risch, and J. C. Gillin (1992). Controlled trial of bright light for nonseasonal major depressive disorders. *Biol. Psychiatry* 31: 119–34.

11. Clodore, M., J. Floret, et al. (1990). Psychophysiological effects of early morning bright light exposure in young adults. *Psychoneuroendocrinology* 15 (3): 193–205.

12. National Sleep Foundation (1998). *Women and Sleep Poll.* Los Angeles: National Sleep Foundation.

13. Park, S. J., and H. Tokura (1999). Bright light exposure during the daytime affects circadian rhythms of urinary melatonin and salivary immunoglobulin A. *Chronobiol. Int.* 16 (3): 359–71.

14. Campbell, S. S., D. Dawson, et al. (1993). Alleviation of sleep maintenance insomnia with timed exposure to bright light. *J. Am. Geriatr. Soc.* 41 (8): 829–36.

15. Vasile, R. G., G. Sachs, et al. (1997). Changes in regional cerebral blood flow following light treatment for seasonal affective disorder: Responders versus nonresponders. *Biol. Psychiatry* 42 (11): 1000–5.

16. Wirz-Justice, A., P. Graw, et al. (1996). Natural light treatment of seasonal affective disorder. *J. Affect. Disord.* 37: 109–20.

17. Christensen, L., and L. Pettijohn (2001). Mood and carbohydrate cravings. *Appetite* 36: 137–45.

18. Ibid.

19. Wurtman, J. J., A. Brzezinski, et al. (1989). Effect of nutrient intake on premenstrual depression. *Am. J. Obstet. Gynecol.* 161 (5): 1228–34.

20. Ibid.

21. Yang, Z. J., M. Koseki, et al. (1996). Eating-related increase of dopamine concentration in the LHA with oronasal stimulation. *Am. J. Physiol.* 270 (2 Pt 2): R315–8.

22. Ibid.

23. Wirz-Justice, Graw, et al. 1996.

24. Pinchasov, B. B., A. M. Shurgaja, et al. (2000). Mood and energy regulation in seasonal and nonseasonal depression before and after midday treatment with physical exercise or bright light. *Psychiatry Res.* 94 (1): 29–42.

25. Wang, G. J., N. D. Volkow, J. Logan, N. R. Pappas, C. T. Wong, W. Zhu, N. Netusil, and J. S. Fowler (2001). Brain dopamine and obesity. *Lancet* 357 (9253): 354–7. *Note:* There is a possibility that people with clinically severe obesity have few dopamine receptors because they have been flooding their bodies with dopamine from frequent eating, resulting in down-regulation of the receptors. The investigators did not believe this to be the case, however.

26. Bylesjo, E. I., K. Boman, et al. (1996). Obesity treated with phototherapy: Four case studies. *Int. J. Eat. Disord.* 20 (4): 443–6.

27. Braun, D. L., S. R. Sunday, et al. (1999). Bright light therapy decreases winter binge frequency in women with bulimia nervosa: A double-blind, placebo-controlled study. *Compr. Psychiatry* 40 (6): 442–8.

28. Zeitzer, J. M., D. J. Dijk, R. Kronauer, E. Brown, and C. Czeisler (2000). Sensitivity of the human circadian pacemaker to nocturnal light: Melatonin phase resetting and suppression. *J. Physiol.* (Lond) 526: 695–702.

29. Nagayama, H., M. Sasaki, et al. (1991). Atypical depressive symptoms possibly predict responsiveness to phototherapy in seasonal affective disorder. *J. Affect. Disord.* 23 (4): 185–9.

Chapter 5

1. Report from Healthy People 2000.

2. Hellstrom, G., and N. G. Wahlgren (1993). Physical exercise increases middle cerebral artery blood flow velocity. *Neurosurg. Rev.* 16 (2): 151–6.

3. Molloy, D. W., D. A. Beerschoten, M. J. Borrie, R. G. Crilly, and R. D. Cape (1998). Acute effects of exercise on neuropsychological function in elderly subjects. *J. Am. Geriatr. Soc.* 36 (1): 29–33.

4. Tate, Andrew K., and Steven J. Petruzzello (1995). Varying the intensity of acute exercise: Implications for changes in affect. *J. Sports Med. Phys. Fitness* 35: 295–302.

5. Thayer, R. E. (1987). Energy, tiredness, and tension effects of a sugar snack versus moderate exercise. *J. Pers. Soc. Psychol.* 52: 119–25.

6. Dey, Sangita (1994). Physical exercise as a novel antidepressant agent: Possible role of serotonin receptor subtypes. *Physiology and Behavior* 55: 323–9.

7. Dishman, R. K. (1997). Brain monoamines, exercise, and behavioral stress: Animal models. *Med. Sci. Sports Exerc.* 29: 63–74.

8. Weicker, H., and H. K. Struder (2001). Influence of exercise on serotonergic neuromodulation in the brain. *Amino Acids* 20 (1): 35–47.

9. Moses, J., A. Steptoe, et al. (1989). The effects of exercise training on mental well-being in the normal population: A controlled trial. *J. Psychosom. Res.* 33 (1): 47–61.

10. Dey 1994.

11. Rejeski, W. J., A. Thompson, et al. (1992). Acute exercise: Buffering psychosocial stress responses in women. *Health Psychol.* 11 (6): 355–62.

12. Roth, D. L. (1989). Acute emotional and psychophysiological effects of aerobic exercise. *Psychophysiology* 26 (5): 593–602.

13. Harte, J. L., and G. H. Eifert (1995). The effects of running, environment, and attentional focus on athletes' catecholamine and cortisol levels and mood. *Psychophysiology* 32: 49–54.

14. Partonen, T., S. Leppamaki, et al. (1998). Randomized trial of physical exercise alone or combined with bright light on mood and health-related quality of life. *Psychol. Med.* 28 (6): 1359–64, p. 1363. The light in the dim room was from 200 to 400 lux. The light in the bright room ranged from 2,500 to 4,000 lux. Four thousand lux is only 1/10th of the amount of light outdoors on a sunny day.

15. Wolfe, R. R. (1998). Fat metabolism in exercise. *Adv. Exp. Med. Biol.* 441: 147–56.

16. Lee, I. M., K. M. Rexrode, N. R. Cook, J. E. Manson, and J. E. Buring (2001). Physical activity and coronary heart disease in women: Is "no pain, no gain" passé? *JAMA* 285: 1447–54.

17. Moradi, T., O. Nyren, M. Zack, C. Magnusson, I. Persson, and H. O. Adami (2000). Breast cancer risk and lifetime leisure-time and occupational physical activity (Sweden). *Cancer Causes Control* 11: 523–31.

18. Exercise lengthens life of postmenopausal women (1997). *Int. J. Fertil. Womens Med.* 42: 182–3.

Chapter 6

1. Benton, D., J. Fordy, and J. Haller (1995). The impact of long-term vitamin supplementation on cognitive functioning. *Psychopharmacology* (Berl) 117: 298–305.

2. Benton, D., Rebecca Griffiths, and J. Haller (1997). Thiamine supplementation, mood, and cognitive functioning. *Psychopharmacology* 129: 66–71.

3. Smidt, L. J., F. M. Cremin, et al. (1991). Influence of thiamine supplementation on the health and general well-being of an elderly Irish population with marginal thiamine deficiency. *J. Gerontol.* 46 (1): M16–22.

4. Bell, I. R., J. S. Edman, et al. (1992). Brief communication. Vitamin B_1, B_2, and B_6 augmentation of tricyclic antidepressant treatment in geriatric depression with cognitive dysfunction. *J. Am. Coll. Nutr.* 11 (2): 159–63.

5. Ibid.

6. Bailey, A. L., S. Maisey, S. Southon, A. J. Wright, P. M. Finglas, and R. A. Fulcher (1997). Relationships between micronutrient intake and biochem-

ical indicators of nutrient adequacy in a "free-living" elderly UK population. *Br. J. Nutr.* 77: 225–42.

7. Demisch, L., and P. Kaczmarczyk (1991). Tryptophan metabolism in healthy subjects: Influence of pyridoxine after single or repeated administrations. *Adv. Exp. Med. Biol.* 294: 519–22.

8. For an overview of how omega-3 fatty acids influence your mood, read *The Omega Diet*, by Dr. Artemis Simopoulos and Jo Robinson (the coauthor of *When Your Body Gets the Blues*). New York: HarperCollins, 1999.

9. Benton, Fordy, and Haller 1995.

10. Van Rensburg, J., and P. Marthinus (1988). Treatment of depression with cognitive-behaviour therapy and vitamin B$_6$. Unpublished data.

11. Munoz-Hoyos, A., I. Amoros-Rodriguez, et al. (1996). Pineal response after pyridoxine test in children. *J. Neural. Transm. Gen. Sect.* 103 (7): 833–42.

12. Doll, H., S. Brown, et al. (1989). Pyridoxine (vitamin B$_6$) and the premenstrual syndrome: A randomized crossover trial. *J. R. Coll. Gen. Pract.* 39 (326): 364–8.

13. Carbajal, A., C. Nunez, et al. (1996). Energy intake as a determinant factor of vitamin status in healthy young women. *Int. J. Vitam. Nutr. Res.* 66 (3): 227–31.

14. Alpert, J. E., and M. Fava (1997). Nutrition and depression: The role of folate. *Nutrition Reviews* 55 (5): 145–9.

15. Coppen, A., and J. Bailey (2000). Enhancement of the antidepressant action of fluoxetine by folic acid: A randomized, placebo controlled trial. *J. Affect. Disord.* 60 (2): 121–30, p. 122.

16. Ibid.

17. Guaraldi, G. P., M. Fava, F. Mazzi, and P. la Greca (1993). An open trial of methyltetrahydrofolate in elderly depressed patients. *Ann. Clin. Psychiatry* 5: 101–5.

18. Botez, M. I., S. N. Young, J. Bachevalier, and S. Gauthier (1982). Effect of folic acid and vitamin B$_{12}$ deficiencies on 5-hydroxyindoleacetic acid [a metabolite of serotonin] in human cerebrospinal fluid. *Ann. Neurol.* 12: 479–84.

19. Rimm, E. B., W. C. Willett, et al. (1998). Folate and vitamin B$_6$ from diet and supplements in relation to risk of coronary heart disease among women. *JAMA* 279 (5): 359–64.

20. Stryd, R. P., T. J. Gilbertson, et al. (1979). A seasonal variation study of 25-hydroxyvitamin D$_3$ serum levels in normal humans. *J. Clin. Endocrinol. Metab.* 48 (5): 771–5.

21. Lansdowne, A. T., and S. C. Provost (1998). Vitamin D$_3$ enhances mood in healthy subjects during winter. *Psychopharmacology* (Berl) 135 (4): 319–23.

22. Matsuoka, L. Y., L. Ide, J. Wortsman, J. A. MacLaughlin, and M. F. Holick (1987). Sunscreens suppress cutaneous vitamin D$_3$ synthesis. *J. Clin. Endocrinol. Metab.* 64 (6): 1165–8.

23. Vieth, R. (1999). Vitamin D supplementation, 25-hydroxyvitamin D concentrations, and safety. *Am. J. Clin. Nutr.* 69: 842–56.

24. Norman, A. W. (1998). Sunlight, season, skin pigmentation, vitamin D, and 25-hydroxyvitamin D: Integral components of the vitamin D endocrine system. *Am. J. Clin. Nutr.* 67 (6): 1108–10.

25. Webb, A. R., L. Kline, et al. (1988). Influence of season and latitude on the cutaneous synthesis of vitamin D$_3$: Exposure to winter sunlight in Boston and Edmonton will not promote vitamin D$_3$ synthesis in human skin. *J. Clin. Endocrinol. Metab.* 67 (2): 373–8.

26. Benton, D., and R. Cook (1990). Selenium supplementation improves mood in a double-blind crossover trial. *Psychopharmacology* 102 (4): 549–50.

27. Castano, A., A. Ayala, J. A. Rodriguez-Gomez, A. J. Herrera, J. Cano, and A. Machado (1997). Low selenium diet increases the dopamine turnover in prefrontal cortex of the rat. *Neurochem. Int.* 30 (6): 549–55.

28. Clark, L. C., G. F. Combs Jr., et al. (1996). Effects of selenium supplementation for cancer prevention in patients with carcinoma of the skin: A randomized controlled trial. Nutritional prevention of cancer study group. *JAMA* 276 (24): 1957–63.

Chapter 7

1. Karakucuk, S., G. Ertugrul Mirza, et al. (1995). Selenium concentrations in serum, lens, and aqueous humour of patients with senile cataract. *Acta. Ophthalmol. Scand.* 73 (4): 329–32. (*Note:* In animals, an overdose of selenium has been associated with a *higher* risk of cataracts. As indicated earlier in the book, your total selenium intake should not exceed 400 micrograms.)

2. Head, K. A. (2001). Natural therapies for ocular disorders (part 2): Cataracts and glaucoma. *Altern. Med. Rev.* 6 (2): 141–66.

3. Mares-Perlman, J. A., B. J. Lyle, R. Klein, A. I. Fisher, W. E. Brady, G. M. VandenLangenberg, J. N. Trabulsi, and M. Palta (2000). Vitamin supplement use and incident cataracts in a population-based study. *Arch. Ophthalmol.* 118: 1556–63.

4. Meesters, Y., D. G. Beersma, et al. (1999). Prophylactic treatment of seasonal affective disorder (SAD) by using light visors: Bright white or infrared light? *Biol. Psychiatry* 46 (2): 239–46.

5. Avery, D. H., M. A. Bolte, et al. (1994). Dawn simulation compared with a dim red signal in the treatment of winter depression. *Biol. Psychiatry* 36 (3): 180–8.

6. Wang, S. Q., R. Setlow, M. Berwick, D. Polsky, A. A. Marghoob, A. W. Kopf, and R. S. Bart (2001). Ultraviolet A and melanoma: A review. *J. Am. Acad. Dermatol.* 44: 837–46.

7. Partonen, T., and J. Lonnqvist (2000). Bright light improves vitality and alleviates distress in healthy people. *J. Affect. Disord.* 57 (1–3): 55–61.

8. Heschong, L., and D. Mahone, et al. (1999). *Skylighting and Retail Sales.* Fair Oaks, Calif.: Heschong Mahone Group.

9. Pacchierotti, C., S. Iapichino, et al. (2001). Melatonin in psychiatric disorders: A review on the melatonin involvement in psychiatry. *Front. Neuroendocrinol.* 22 (1): 18–32.

10. Labbate, L. A., B. Lafer, et al. (1994). Side effects induced by bright light treatment for seasonal affective disorder. *J. Clin. Psychiatry* 55 (5): 189–91.

11. Heschong, L. and D. Mahone, et al. (1999). *Daylighting in Schools.* Page 29. Fair Oaks, Calif.: Heschong Mahone Group.

12. Campbell, S. S., D. F. Kripke, J. C. Gillin, and J. C. Hrubovcak (1998). Exposure to light in healthy elderly subjects and Alzheimer's patients. *Physiol. Behav.* 42: 141–4.

13. Satlin, A., L. Volicer, V. Ross, L. Herz, and S. Campbell (1992). Bright light treatment of behavioral and sleep disturbances in patients with Alzheimer's disease. *Am. J. Psychiatry* 149: 1028–32.

Chapter 8

1. Ekkekakis, P., E. E. Hall, et al. (2000). Walking in (affective) circles: Can short walks enhance affect? *J. Behav. Med.* 23 (3): 245–75.

2. Shephard, R. J., S. Thomas, and I. Weller. (1991). The Canadian home fitness test: 1991 update. *Sports Medicine* 1: 359.

Chapter 10

1. Refer to the notes for chapter 7 for specific references.

Index

Underscored page references indicate boxed text. **Boldface** references indicate illustrations.

A

All-or-nothing thinking, avoiding, 148
Alternative therapies, for Body Blues, 11–12, 12, 42–43
Andropause, 35
Antidepressant cocktail. *See* LEVITY formula
Antidepressants
  for Body Blues, 8–9, 11
  folic acid taken with, 91
  LEVITY program combined with, 20, 142
  vs. light therapy, 62
  Prozac as (*see* Prozac)
  relapse rate after discontinuing, 51
  vitamin B$_1$ and, 87
Audiobooks, for walking, 127, 169

B

Baby blues, symptoms of, 32
Beck Depression Inventory (BDI), Body Blues overlooked by, 12
Birth defects, folic acid for preventing, 92
Body Blues
  alternative remedies for, 11–12, 12, 42–43
  beginning of, 31
  after childbirth, 32–33, 33

in children, 21
diagnosis of, 12
genes influencing, 34
hormones affecting
  estrogen, 9–10, 23–25
  progesterone, 25–27
  testosterone, 27–29
LEVITY program for (*see* LEVITY program)
lifestyle influencing, 34
medications for, 11, 42
in men, 21, 35
menopausal symptoms as, 5, 8
during menstrual cycle, 29, **30**
19th-century treatment of, 8
during perimenopause, 20, 21, 33
personal story of, 5–7
PMS as, 5, 8, 21, 27
postpartum depression as, 5, 8
quiz for diagnosing, 14–17
  flow chart on, **18–19**
  questions and answers about, 17, 20–21
seasonal affective disorder as, 5, 8, 21
serotonin and, 9–10
stress triggering, 75–76
symptom log for
  blank, **38–39**
  directions for using, 36
  example of, **37**
symptoms of, 3–5

About the Authors

Marie-Annette Brown, Ph.D., R.N., is a professor in the School of Nursing at the University of Washington who is involved in research, teaching, and clinical practice. Dr. Brown has lectured widely and published more than 60 scientific papers. She is nationally certified as a family and psychiatric/mental health nurse practitioner and provides primary care at the University of Washington Women's Health Care Clinic.

Jo Robinson is a *New York Times* best-selling author from Vashon Island, Washington, who specializes in books on mental health and nutrition. She is the coauthor of 11 popular books, including *Getting the Love You Want, Hot Monogamy,* and *The Omega Diet.* She collaborated with Dr. Brown in the design of the LEVITY study.